Frozen Section Library

Series Editor
Philip T. Cagle, MD
Houston, Texas, USA

Frozen Section Library: Liver, Extrahepatic Biliary Tree and Gallbladder

Edited by

Rhonda K. Yantiss, MD

*Weill Medical College of Cornell University,
New York, NY, USA*

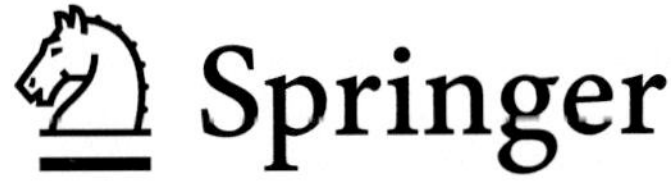

Editor
Rhonda K. Yantiss, MD
Department of Pathology and Laboratory Medicine
Weill Medical College of Cornell University
New York, NY, USA
rhy2001@med.cornell.edu

ISSN 1868-4157   e-ISSN 1868-4165
ISBN 978-1-4614-0042-4   e-ISBN 978-1-4614-0043-1
DOI 10.1007/978-1-4614-0043-1
Springer New York Dordrecht Heidelberg London

Library of Congress Control Number: 2011931087

Printed on acid-free paper

Springer is part of Springer Science+Business Media (www.springer.com)

Series Preface

For over 100 years, the frozen section has been utilized as a tool for the rapid diagnosis of specimens while a patient is undergoing surgery, usually under general anesthesia, as a basis for making immediate treatment decisions. Frozen section diagnosis is often a challenge for the pathologist who must render a diagnosis that has crucial import for the patient in a minimal amount of time. In addition to the need for rapid recall of differential diagnoses, there are many pitfalls and artifacts that add to the risk of frozen section diagnosis that are not present with permanent sections of fully processed tissues that can be examined in a more leisurely fashion. Despite the century-long utilization of frozen sections, most standard pathology textbooks, both general and subspecialty, largely ignore the topic of frozen sections. Few textbooks have ever focused exclusively on frozen section diagnosis and those textbooks that have done so are now out-of-date and have limited illustrations.

The Frozen Section Library Series is meant to provide convenient, user-friendly handbooks for each organ system to expedite use in the rushed frozen section situation. These books are small and lightweight, copiously color illustrated with images of actual frozen sections, highlighting pitfalls, artifacts, and differential diagnosis. The advantages of a series of organ-specific handbooks, in addition to the ease-of-use and manageable size, are that (1) a series allows more comprehensive coverage of more diagnoses, both common and rare, than a single volume that tries to highlight a limited number of diagnoses for each organ and (2) a series allows more detailed insight by permitting experienced authorities to emphasize the peculiarities of frozen section for each organ system.

As a handbook for practicing pathologists, these books will be indispensable aids to diagnosis and avoiding dangers in one of the most challenging situations that pathologists encounter. Rapid consideration of differential diagnoses and how to avoid traps caused by frozen section artifacts are emphasized in these handbooks. A series of concise, easy-to-use, well-illustrated handbooks alleviates the often frustrating and time-consuming, sometimes futile, process of searching through bulky textbooks that are unlikely to illustrate or discuss pathologic diagnoses from the perspective of frozen sections in the first place. Tables and charts will provide guidance for differential diagnosis of various histologic patterns. Touch preparations, which are used for some organs such as central nervous system or thyroid more often than others, are appropriately emphasized and illustrated according to the need for each specific organ.

This series is meant to benefit practicing surgical pathologists, both community and academic, and to pathology residents and fellows; and also to provide valuable perspectives to surgeons, surgery residents, and fellows who must rely on frozen section diagnosis by their pathologists. Most of all, we hope that this series contributes to the improved care of patients who rely on the frozen section to help guide their treatment.

Philip T. Cagle, MD

Preface

Despite many recent advances in ancillary techniques, intraoperative pathology consultation remains one of the most diagnostically and technically challenging areas of surgical pathology. Frozen sections are usually performed while the patient is under general anesthesia and play an important role in making immediate treatment decisions. Unfortunately, most standard pathology textbooks largely ignore the topic of frozen section, including the pitfalls and artifacts associated with frozen section preparation, and the value of gross examination of surgical resection specimens is no longer emphasized in many training programs.

The *Frozen Section of the Liver, Extrahepatic Biliary Tree, and Gallbladder,* is a volume in the *Frozen Section Library Series.* The book is divided into seven chapters, each of which discusses the clinical context in which a frozen section consultation may be requested. The chapters emphasize gross characteristics of liver and biliary disease, address common questions pathologists must answer during frozen section examination, and discuss pitfalls encountered during frozen section analysis. Recommendations regarding specimen handling are also provided.

We hope that this monograph satisfies the need for practical guidelines for the handling and interpretation of resection specimens and facilitates communications between surgical pathologists and our surgical colleagues.

New York, NY

Rhonda K. Yantiss
Nicole C. Panarelli

Contents

Contributor

Nicole C. Panarelli, MD
Department of Pathology and Laboratory Medicine
Weill Medical College of Cornell University
New York, NY, USA

Chapter 1
Intraoperative Evaluation of Primary Hepatocellular Tumors

INTRODUCTION

Hepatocellular tumors show characteristic clinical and radiographic features that aid their classification and needle biopsy evaluation is generally limited to those with unusual features. Thus, intraoperative classification is reserved for situations in which an unsuspected liver nodule is encountered during organ harvest or surgical exploration for indications unrelated to hepatic disease. However, preoperative needle biopsy of liver tumors may seed the needle tract, particularly when using wide-bore or cutting needles, so some surgeons still use frozen section analysis to make a primary diagnosis [1–4]. Intraoperative frozen section analysis is also used to assess the adequacy of surgical resection for hepatic tumors. Different types of hepatocellular tumors are not always treated similarly, so their correct classification is important to immediate patient care. Thus, pathologists should be aware of the spectrum of primary hepatocellular lesions that may be encountered during intraoperative consultation (Table 1.1).

ASSESSMENT OF MARGINS

The assessment of resection margins for hepatocellular tumors is relatively straightforward, but requires an understanding of the indications for, and type of, surgical procedure performed. Most liver tumor surgeries result in partial resection specimens, in which case the most important resection margin is that of the hepatic parenchyma. The extent of resection is largely determined by the tumor location within the liver and reflects the vascular supply to the hepatic segments (Fig. 1.1). The parenchymal resec-

1

R.K. Yantiss (ed.), *Frozen Section Library: Liver, Extrahepatic Biliary Tree and Gallbladder*, Frozen Section Library, DOI 10.1007/978-1-4614-0043-1_1,
© Springer Science+Business Media, LLC 2011

TABLE 1.1 Gross and histologic features of hepatocellular tumors.

Tumor	Background liver	Gross features	Histologic features
Hepatocellular carcinoma	Fibrotic or cirrhotic	Pale brown or green Solitary or multiple	Infiltrative of adjacent liver Trabecular, acinar, pseudoglandular architecture Intracellular bile Increased nuclear to cytoplasmic ratio Prominent nucleoli Mitotic figures readily identified
Fibrolamellar hepatocellular carcinoma	Normal	Pale brown with fibrous septa Solitary	Cell clusters enmeshed in dense collagen Voluminous eosinophilic cytoplasm Eosinophilic cytoplasmic "pale bodies" Small intracytoplasmic hyaline globules Macronucleoli
Hepatocellular adenoma	Normal	Pale brown, yellow, or bile-stained May be hemorrhagic Subcapsular	Sheets of normal-appearing hepatocytes Fibrous septa, but no portal tracts Thickened cell plates "Naked" blood vessels in parenchyma
Focal nodular hyperplasia	Normal	Pale brown with fibrous septa Well-circumscribed but unencapsulated	Nodules of normal hepatocytes Radiating septa with ductular proliferation Thickened arteries within fibrous septa

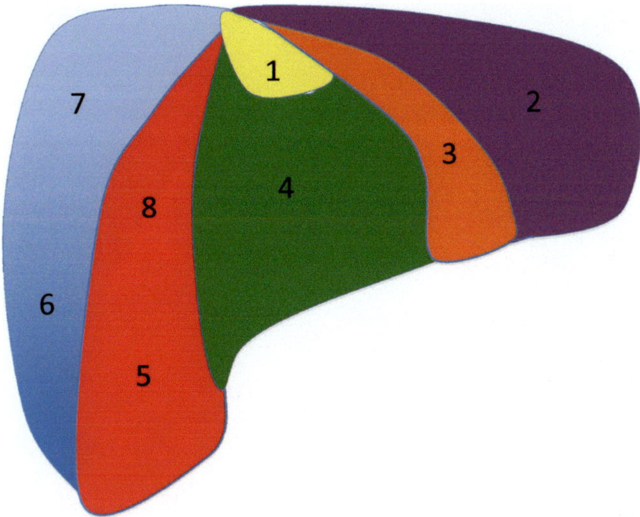

FIG. 1.1 The Couinaud classification scheme divides the liver into eight segments, each of which has its own vascular inflow, vascular outflow, and biliary drainage. Segment 1 is the caudate lobe, which is located posteriorly. The remaining segments are numbered in a clockwise fashion in the frontal plane.

tion margin is readily identifiable as an irregular cauterized tissue edge and should be inked prior to sectioning the liver. Inking of the capsule is not encouraged, since tumor involvement of the capsule does not alter pathologic stage assignment and may cause confusion when interpreting histologic sections. The liver is sectioned perpendicularly to the hepatic margin and a gross photograph of a cross section is obtained to document the relationship between the closest margin and the tumor (Fig. 1.2). Resection margins that are more than 1 cm from the tumor may be taken *en face*, whereas closer margins should be perpendicularly sectioned to include both tumor and the inked resection margin. Bile duct and vascular margins may be evaluated in both partial resection specimens and explanted livers, although pathologists are rarely asked to assess vascular margins intraoperatively. The portal structures are easily recognized on explanted livers, but may not be readily identifiable on resection specimens, thus they should be clearly indicated by the surgeon. Both vascular and bile duct margins are generally examined *en face*

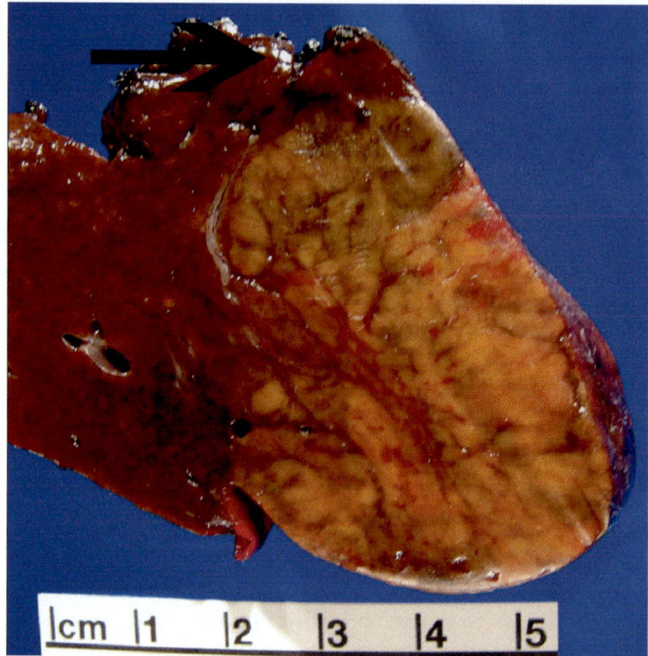

Fig. 1.2 This wedge resection specimen contains a well-circumscribed, pale brown adenoma that is <1 mm from the cauterized, inked resection margin (*arrow*).

HEPATOCELLULAR CARCINOMA

Hepatocellular carcinoma (HCC) is the third leading cause of cancer-related death worldwide, and a major cause of cancer-related morbidity and death in the United States [5, 6]. Unfortunately, HCC is an aggressive type of cancer with a poor prognosis. The mean survival is only 8 months and the 1- and 3-year survival rates are 36 and 17%, respectively [7]. The most important risk factor for HCC development is cirrhosis, which, in the United States, is usually due to chronic hepatitis C virus (HCV) infection, hepatitis B virus infection, or alcoholic liver disease. The incidence of HCC in the United States has more than doubled among individuals 75–79 years of age and increased fourfold among patients 45–49 years of age since the early 1980s, reflecting HCV transmission *via* intravenous drug use and infected blood products [7]. HCC is also a potential complication of nonalcoholic fatty liver disease (NAFLD), which represents a serious health concern among obese patients and likely cause of "cryptogenic" cirrhosis. However, a substantial proportion (15–50%) of patients with HCC does not have any identifiable risk factors [8].

Surgery represents the best treatment option for HCC, although approximately 80% of patients have advanced stage disease or inadequate reserves of hepatic function that preclude them from surgical intervention [7–9]. Patients with compensated liver disease are potentially eligible for partial hepatic resection depending on the anatomic location of the tumor, even if they have cirrhosis. Intraoperative evaluation of these specimens is performed to assess adequacy of excision, so the rough parenchymal resection margin should be inked and perpendicularly sectioned, as previously described. Liver transplantation may be offered to patients with HCC and poor synthetic function secondary to cirrhosis, but only individuals who have small (<5 cm in diameter), solitary lesions or a maximum of three tumors, all of which span no more than 3 cm, are potential candidates for this procedure [7–10]. Explanted livers are not usually submitted for intraoperative consultation. They should, however, be handled in a uniform manner with complete knowledge of the radiographic findings to correlate tumor number, size, and location with the pathologic findings. Explanted livers are weighed, measured, and photographed prior to removal of the portal vein, hepatic artery, and bile duct margins. The entire liver is sliced at 5 mm intervals from superior to inferior in the axial plane, such that each section includes both the right and the left lobes. Photographs of representative cross sections are obtained to document tumor size and location, as well as the underlying medical disease (Fig. 1.3). Representative sections submitted for histologic evaluation include those from the tumor(s) and right, left, and caudate lobes. Other parenchymal nodules spanning 1 cm or more are also sampled, as are any nodules that are distinct from the surrounding parenchyma, regardless of size. Unusual features, including discoloration or bile staining, should prompt histologic assessment (Fig. 1.4). Notably, some patients with HCC may undergo embolization of the tumor prior to transplantation, so pathologists should provide documentation regarding tumor viability (Fig. 1.5).

HCCs may be single or multifocal. They are usually well-circumscribed brown tumors that are discolored compared with the adjacent parenchyma (Fig. 1.6). They may show variable architectural growth patterns. Most commonly, the tumor cells grow in trabeculae composed of cell plates that are at least three cells thick (Fig. 1.7). Some HCCs display an acinar growth pattern with gland-like spaces that contain bile or proteinaceous material, whereas others consist of dense aggregates of tumor cells without

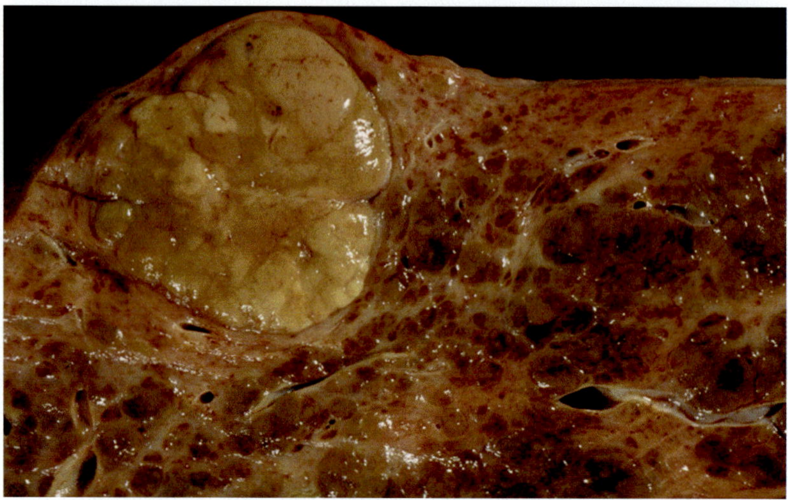

FIG. 1.3 The hepatocellular carcinoma (HCC) in this liver explant is associated with cirrhosis.

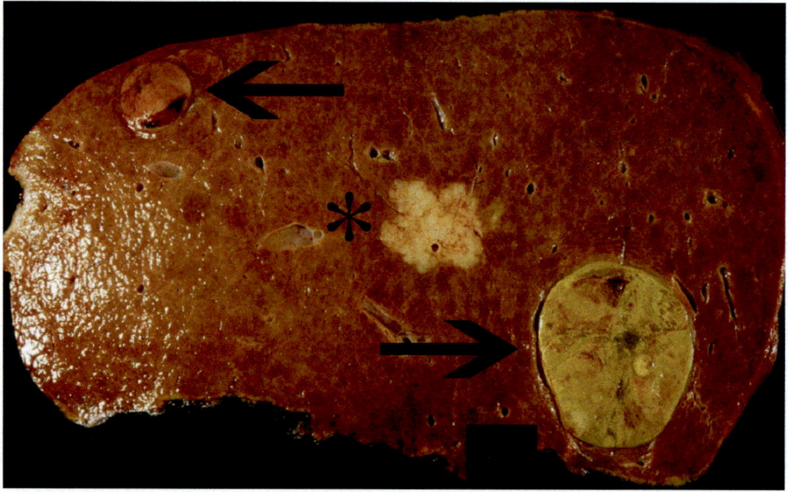

FIG. 1.4 The explanted liver contains three tumor nodules. Two are well-circumscribed and discolored (*arrows*) compared with the background, somewhat fibrotic liver and one is ill-defined (*asterisk*). Both round tumors are HCCs and the irregular white mass is a cholangiocarcinoma.

intervening stroma or apparent vascular spaces (Figs. 1.8 and 1.9). A scirrhous growth pattern is characterized by dense fibrosis around tumor cell nests and single cells and may simulate the appearance of adenocarcinoma, particularly when the neoplastic

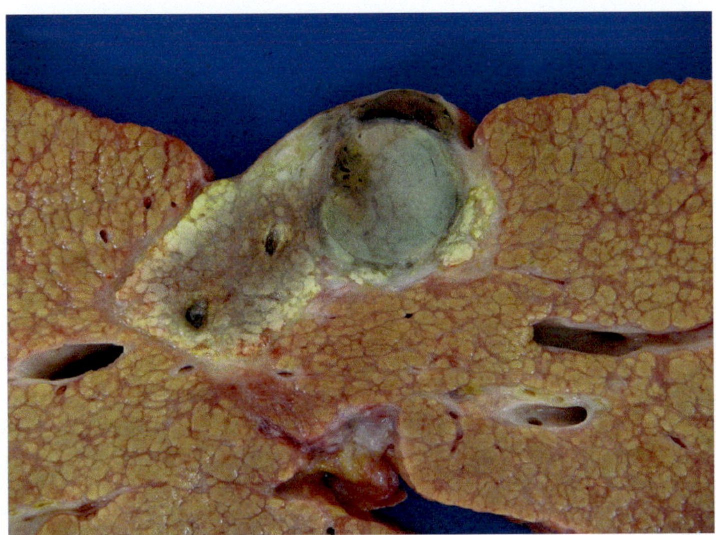

FIG. 1.5 This HCC was embolized prior to transplantation. The tumor is pale green and entirely nonviable. It is surrounded by a rim of necrotic, nonneoplastic hepatic parenchyma.

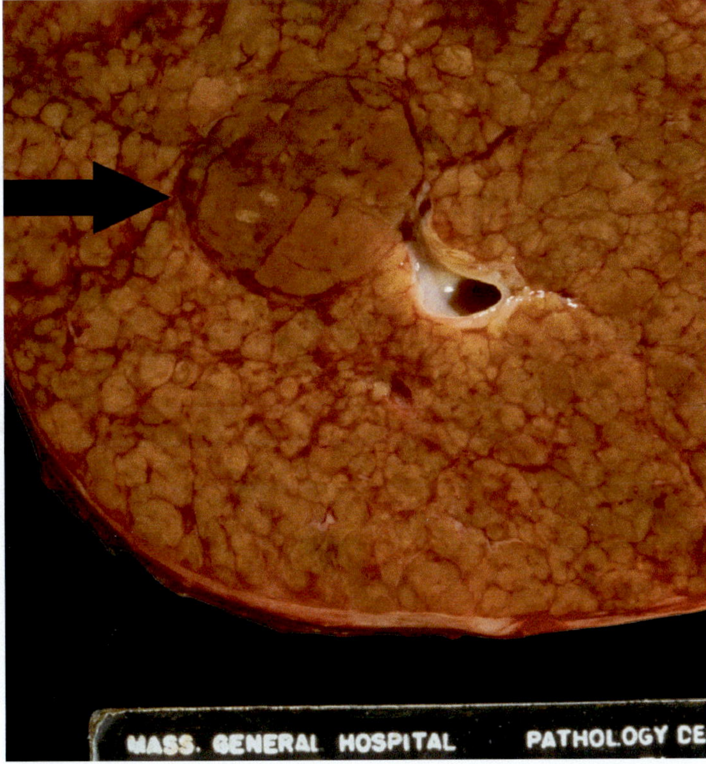

FIG. 1.6 This HCC is a 2.0-cm brown nodule (*arrow*) that is slightly darker than the background cirrhotic liver.

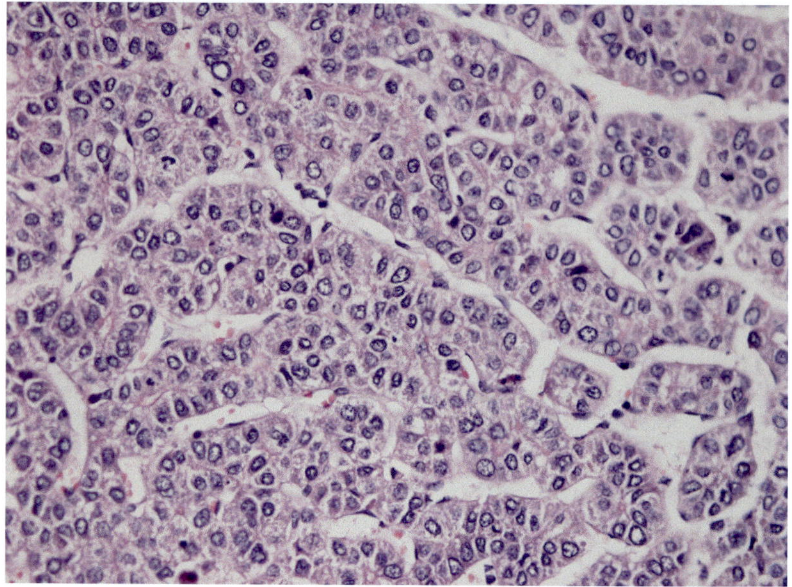

FIG. 1.7 The trabecular growth pattern of HCC shows thickened cell plates surrounded by endothelial cells that line dilated sinusoids.

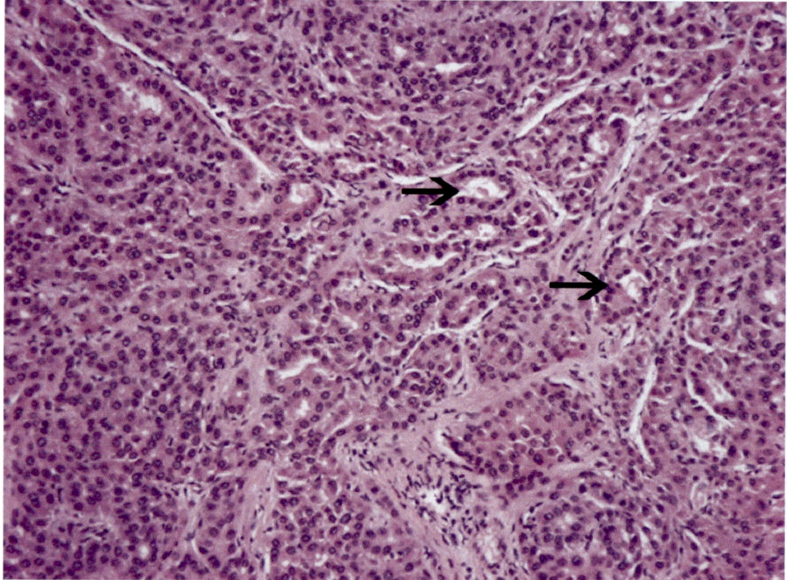

FIG. 1.8 Neoplastic hepatocytes form gland-like ("pseudoacinar") spaces, some of which contain proteinaceous material (*arrows*) (photograph courtesy of Dr. David Klimstra, Memorial Sloan Kettering Cancer Center).

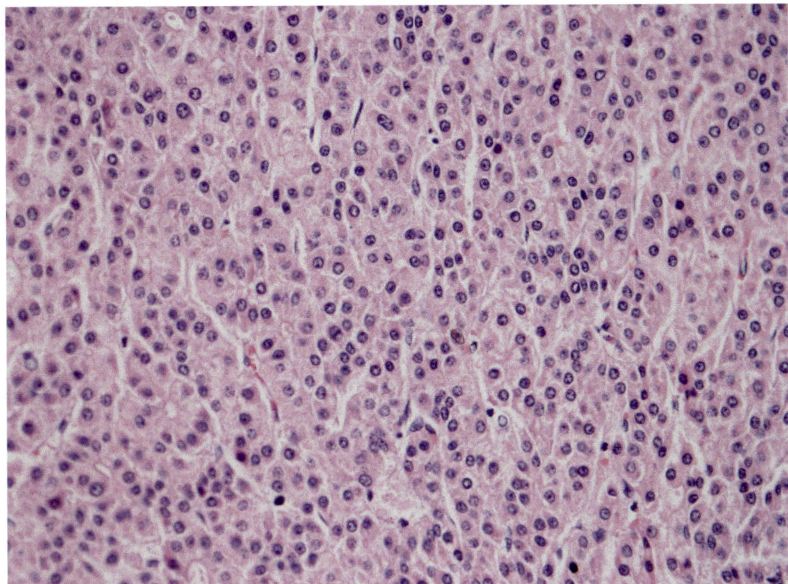

FIG. 1.9 Solid HCCs are composed of sheets of tumor cells without intervening stroma.

cells form pseudoacini (Fig. 1.10). Well-differentiated HCCs display some degree of cytologic atypia, including an increased nuclear to cytoplasmic ratio, irregular nuclear contours, cytoplasmic pseudoinclusions, and variable numbers of mitotic figures (Fig. 1.11). Most high-grade HCCs contain cells with basophilic, rather than eosinophilic, cytoplasm and hyperchromatic angulated nuclei, although large pleomorphic cells and giant cells may be present (Fig. 1.12).

The differential diagnosis of HCC is broad and depends upon the morphologic features of the tumor. At one end of the spectrum, well-differentiated HCC simulates the appearance of a benign hepatocellular tumor, namely hepatocellular adenoma. Both may show minimal cytologic and architectural atypia, although the presence of mitotic activity should lead one to suspect a diagnosis of HCC. Poorly differentiated HCC may be confused with a variety of tumors, including metastastic carcinoma, malignant melanoma, and epithelioid sarcoma. One important point to remember is that, with the exception of fibrolamellar HCC, the vast majority of HCCs develop in association with hepatic fibrosis, whereas metastatic disease in the cirrhotic liver is distinctly uncommon.

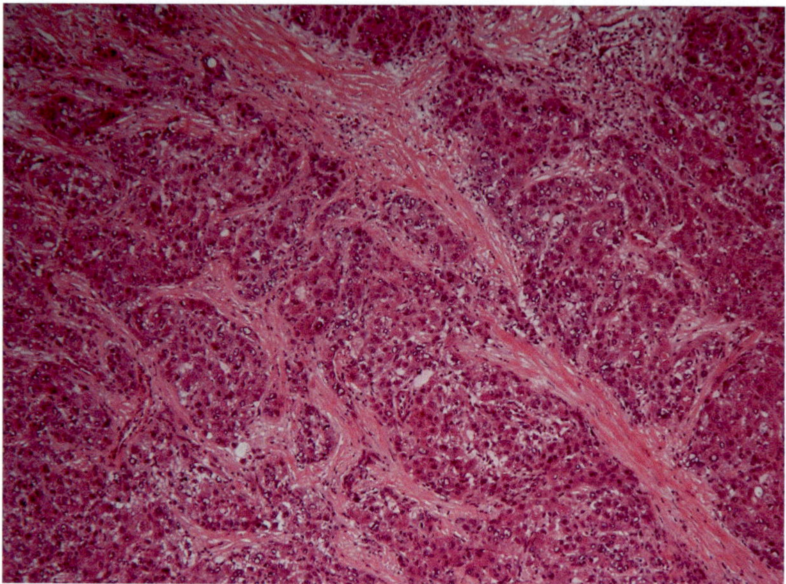

FIG. 1.10 Scirrhous HCCs contain nests of tumor cells separated by dense fibrous bands (photograph courtesy of Dr. David Klimstra, Memorial Sloan Kettering Cancer Center).

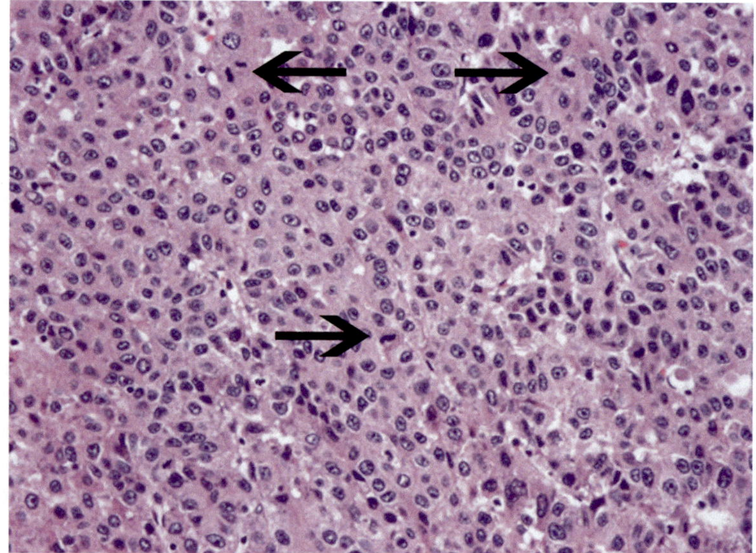

FIG. 1.11 The tumor cells of well-differentiated HCC have an increased nuclear-to-cytoplasmic ratio, irregular nuclear contours, and easily detectable mitotic figures (*arrows*).

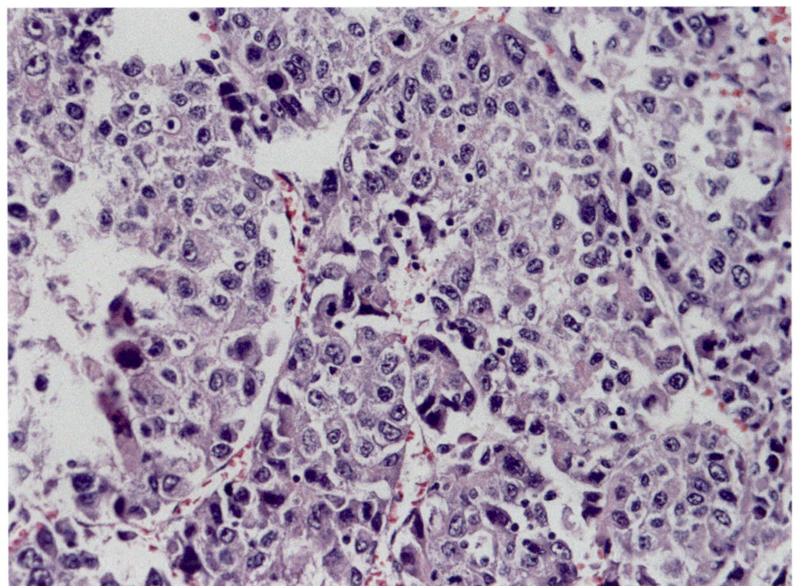

FIG. 1.12   Poorly-differentiated HCCs contain cells with large, hyperchromatic, angulated nuclei, and basophilic cytoplasm.

Fibrolamellar HCC is a subtype of HCC that deserves specific mention. It is a malignancy of young patients that typically occurs in the noncirrhotic liver. Recognizing fibrolamellar HCC at the time of intraoperative evaluation is important since it has a propensity to spread to regional lymph nodes and thus requires a lymph node dissection. Fibrolamellar HCCs characteristically contain a dense central scar corresponding to the presence of paucicellular plates of dense collagen (Figs. 1.13 and 1.14). They consist of tumor cells with voluminous, densely, eosinophilic cytoplasm, faintly eosinophilic inclusions (pale bodies) and hyaline droplets within the cytoplasm, and macronucleoli (Fig. 1.15).

Hepatocellular Adenoma

Hepatocellular adenomas are benign liver tumors that usually develop in young women who take oral contraceptive pills. They may be solitary or multiple in otherwise healthy patients, although multifocal hepatocellular adenomas also occur in patients with metabolic disorders, such as types I and III glycogen storage disease, diabetes mellitus, and beta-thalassemia [11–13]. Hepatocellular adenomas are subcapsular tumors that may be incidentally discovered during abdominal imaging studies

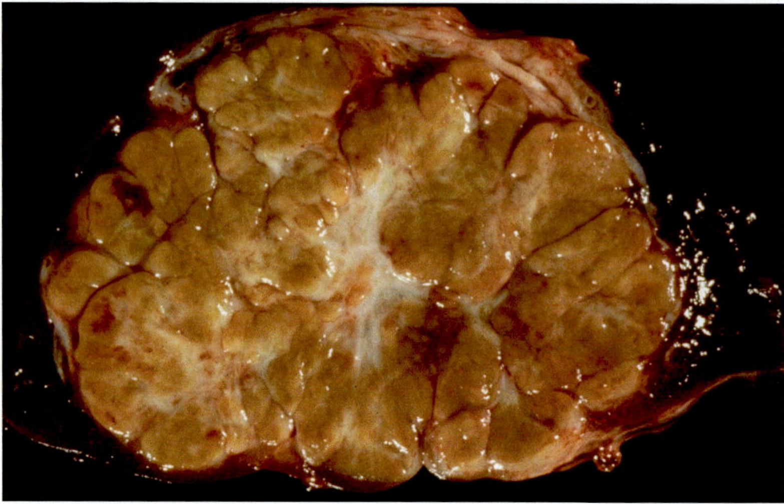

FIG. 1.13 Fibrolamellar HCCs contain a dense central scar and develop in patients without cirrhosis.

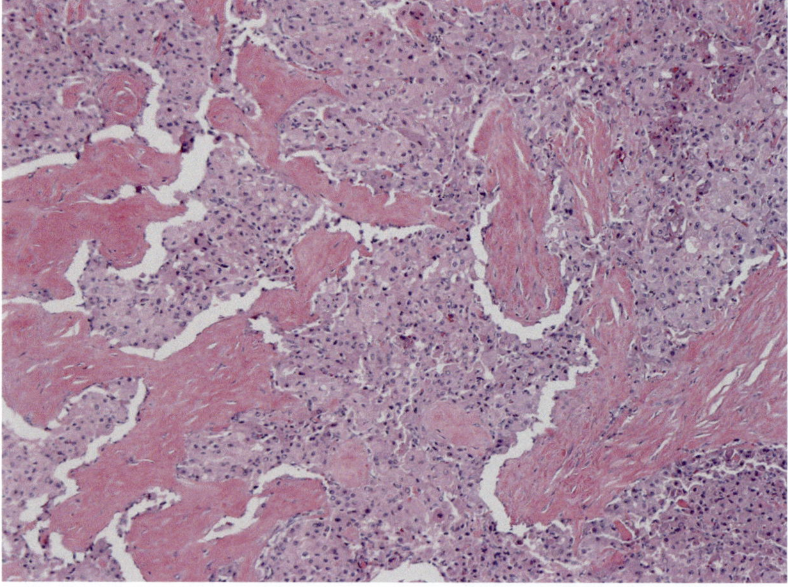

FIG. 1.14 Fibrolamellar HCC is composed of tumor cell aggregates separated by broad, paucicellular fibrous bands. The tumor cells have abundant eosinophilic cytoplasm that is appreciable at low magnification.

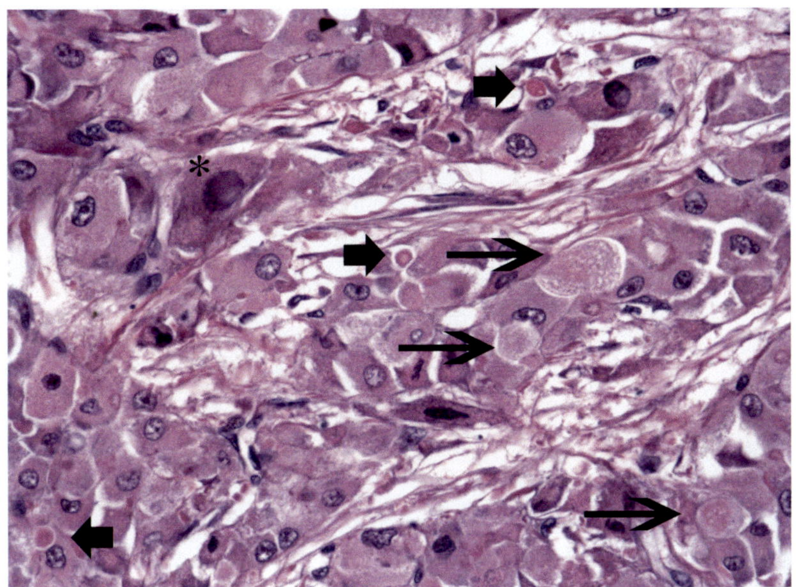

FIG. 1.15 The large, polygonal cells of fibrolamellar HCC contain large nuclei with prominent nucleoli and occasional intranuclear pseudoinclusions (*asterisk*). Faintly eosinophilic cytoplasmic inclusions (*pale bodies*) are present (*long arrows*) as are intracytoplasmic hyaline globules (*block arrows*).

performed for unrelated reasons, or produce abdominal pain as a result of either a mass effect or intratumoral hemorrhage. They have a propensity to spontaneously rupture and bleed, especially under the influence of estrogen (Fig. 1.16). In fact, uncontrolled bleeding into the peritoneal cavity can be life-threatening. These tumors also have potential for malignant transformation in rare cases and, thus, hepatocellular adenomas are often resected once they are discovered.

The distinction between hepatocellular adenoma and HCC is usually straightforward. Both are well-circumscribed, pale brown masses, but most hepatocellular adenomas occur in young women without underlying liver disease (Fig. 1.2). In contrast, HCCs are more common among older men and generally develop in association with cirrhosis (Fig. 1.3). Hepatocellular adenomas are composed of sheets of uniform hepatocytes that are similar in size to adjacent nonlesional hepatocytes, although slightly smaller or larger tumor cells may be identified in some cases (Fig. 1.17). These tumor cells have abundant eosinophilic cytoplasm, but may harbor glycogen or fat, regardless of whether these findings are

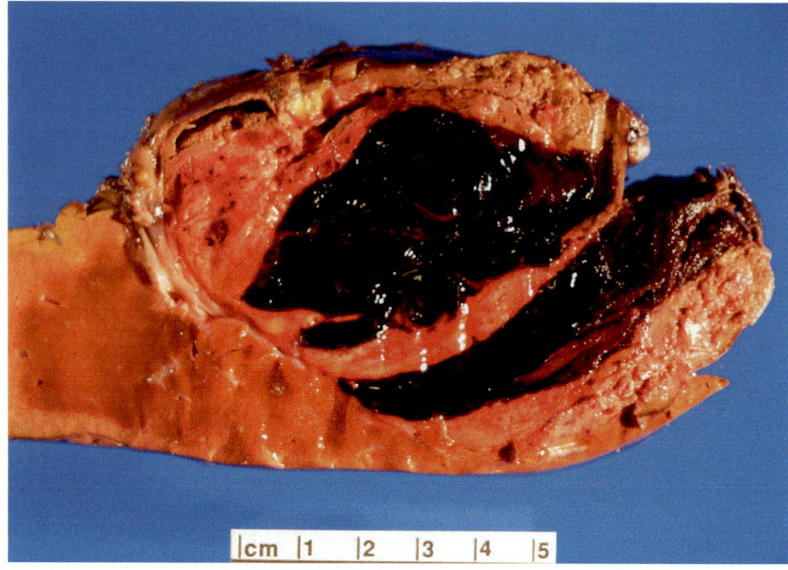

FIG. 1.16 This hepatocellular adenoma was emergently removed due to spontaneous rupture and hemorrhage into the peritoneal cavity. Organizing blood within the tumor extends onto the capsular surface, which is disrupted.

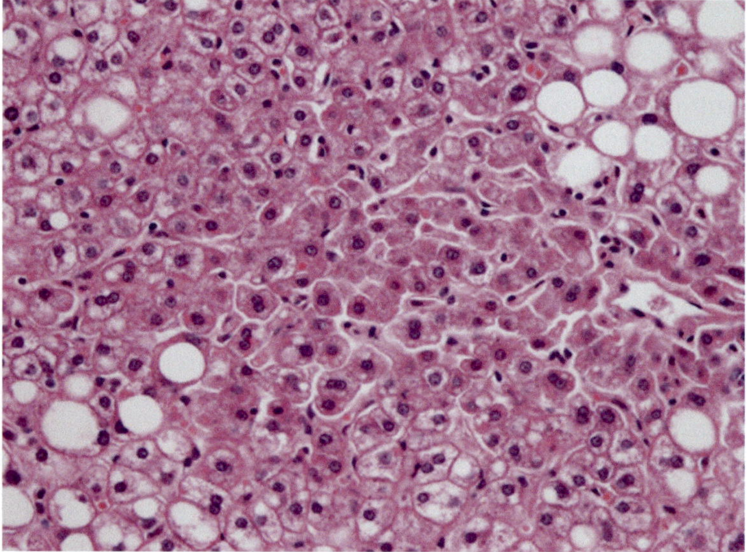

FIG. 1.17 The cells of a hepatocellular adenoma are approximately the same size as the normal hepatocytes and have a low nuclear-to-cytoplasmic ratio. Mitotic figures are absent.

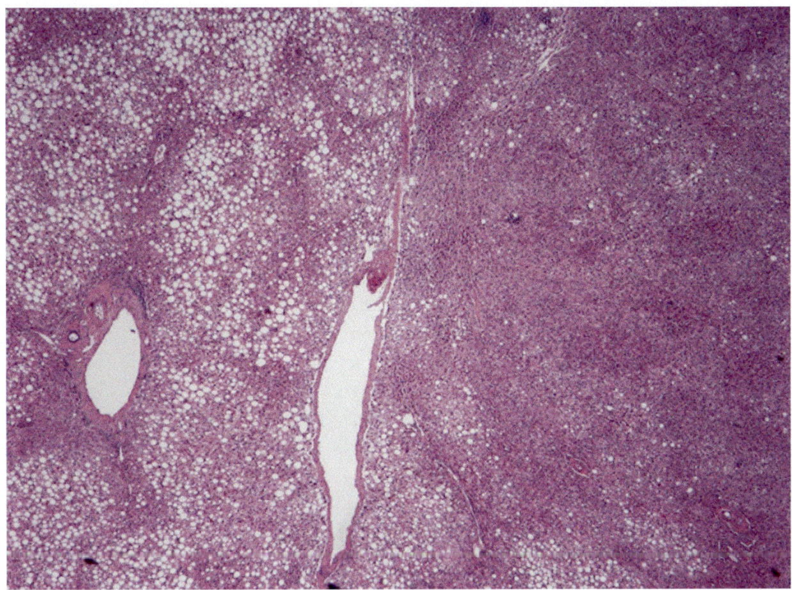

Fɪɢ. 1.18 Hepatocellular adenomas contain sheets of uniform hepato-cytes. The tumor cells (*right*) harbor less fat than the adjacent parenchyma (*left*).

present in adjacent parenchyma (Fig. 1.18). Hepatocellular adenomas contain solitary vessels, many of which have abnormally thick walls (Fig. 1.19). They may also contain broad fibrous septa, but normal portal tracts are lacking. Although the cell plates of hepatocellular adenoma are somewhat expanded, those of HCC are thicker and disorganized with "pseudoglandular" structures and a greater degree of cytologic atypia. The distinction between hepatocellular adenoma and well-differentiated HCC may not be possible based solely upon frozen section analysis. Fortunately, distinguishing between them at the time of surgery is not usually necessary since both are similarly treated by excision. Deferring a diagnosis to permanent sections causes no immediate harm to the patient.

Focal Nodular Hyperplasia

Focal nodular hyperplasia (FNH) is a nonneoplastic tumor that usually occurs in young women unassociated with liver disease. Although it may grow under the influence of estrogen, FNH is not associated with risk of hemorrhage or malignant transformation. Therefore, it is usually managed conservatively with serial imaging

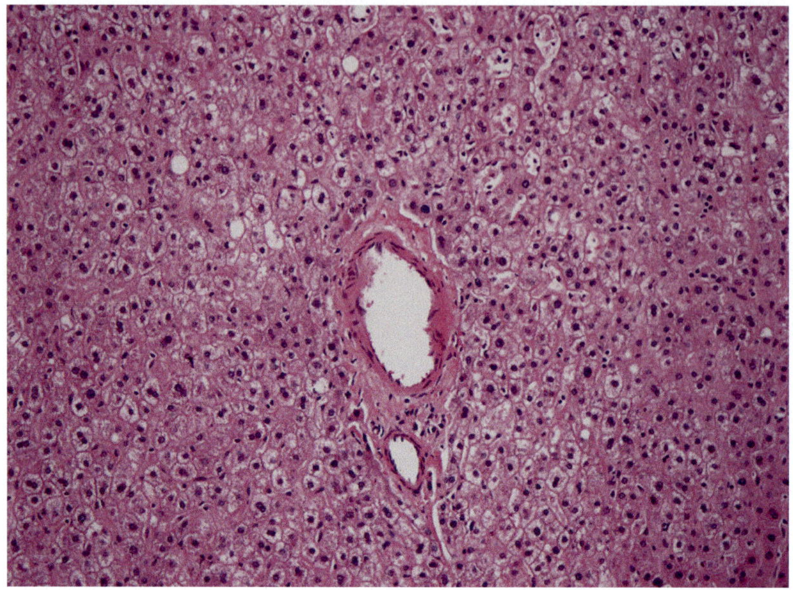

Fig. 1.19 Thick-walled, solitary blood vessels are typical of hepatocellular adenomas.

and discontinuation of oral contraceptive pills [14]. The diagnosis of FNH can be made radiographically owing to the characteristic presence of dense, centrally located fibrosis within the tumor. Histologic evaluation by fine-needle aspiration or needle core biopsy is limited to cases with equivocal imaging findings and is used to exclude the possibility of hepatocellular adenoma or malignancy [14]. Donor livers that contain FNH may be submitted for frozen section evaluation.

Most examples of FNH display a central fibrous scar with radiating bands of fibrosis that extend to the tumor periphery (Fig. 1.20). These tumors contain nodules of normal-appearing hepatocytes surrounded by dense fibrous bands within which one may find proliferating bile ductules and vascular structures (Fig. 1.21). Hepatocytes are arranged in thickened cell plates that form nodules reminiscent of the regenerative nodules of cirrhosis (Fig. 1.22).

The differential diagnosis of FNH includes fibrolamellar HCC and telangiectatic hepatocellular adenoma, both of which may show dense fibrosis and occur in young, noncirrhotic patients. Fibrolamellar HCCs contain broad bands of paucicellular

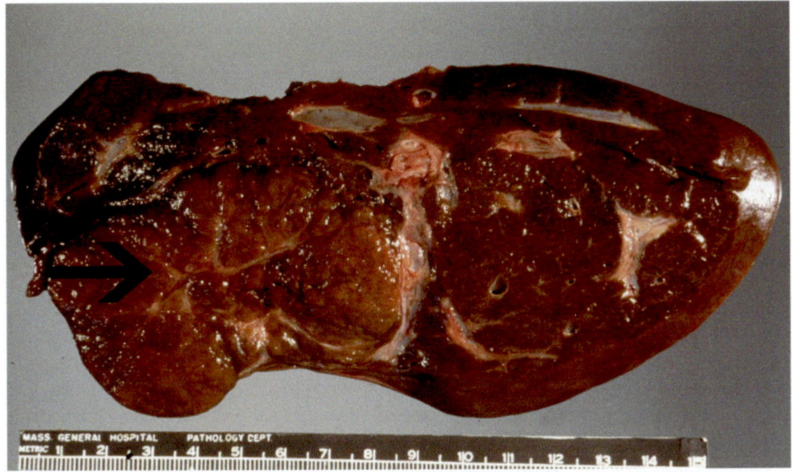

FIG. 1.20 Focal nodular hyperplasia (FNH) simulates the appearance of fibrolamellar HCC. It is unencapsulated with pale brown parenchyma and contains a central scar (*arrow*).

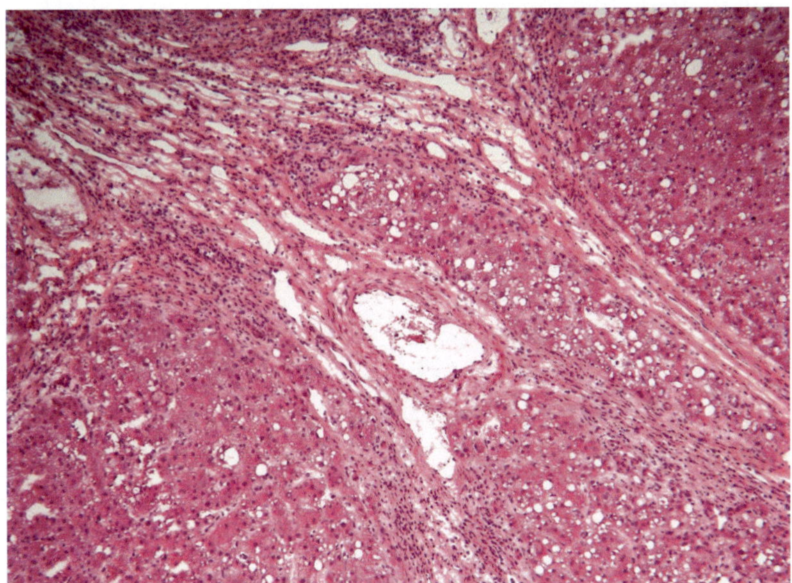

FIG. 1.21 Normal-appearing hepatocytes arranged in thickened cell plates comprise the nodules of FNH (photograph courtesy of Dr. David Klimstra, Memorial Sloan Kettering Cancer Center).

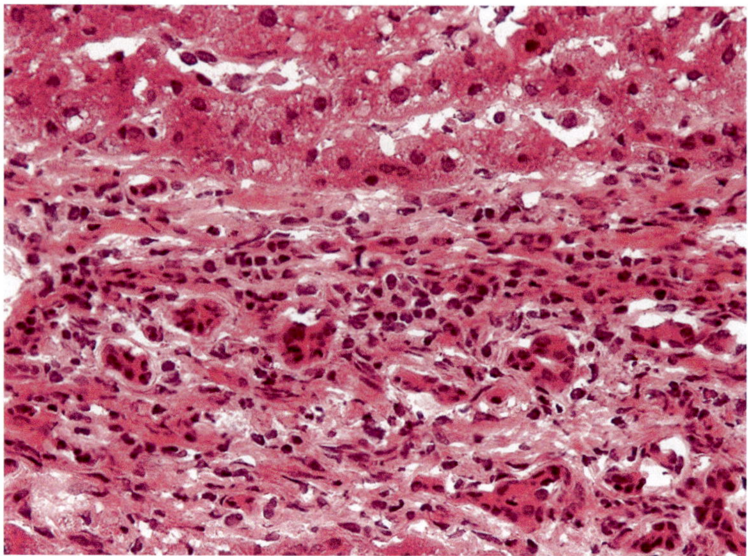

FIG. 1.22 FNH is composed of regenerative nodules of hepatocytes with radiating fibrous septa. The appearance of FNH simulates that of cirrhosis, particularly when evaluation is limited to needle biopsy (photograph courtesy of Dr. David Klimstra, Memorial Sloan Kettering Cancer Center).

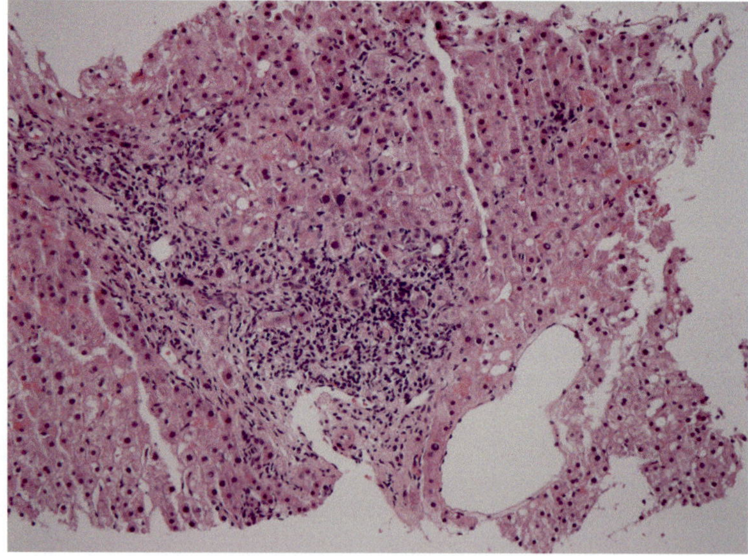

FIG. 1.23 Telangiectatic hepatocellular adenoma contains nodules of proliferating hepatocytes with inflamed fibrous septa and dilated vascular spaces.

collagen that surround individual hepatocytes, whereas the fibrous septa of FNH simulate the appearance of cirrhosis. Fibrolamellar HCCs also contain tumor cells with more abundant, often densely eosinophilic cytoplasm, faintly eosinophilic intracytoplasmic globules, hyaline globules, and Mallory's hyaline. In contrast, FNH is composed of normal-appearing hepatocytes. Telangiectatic hepatocellular adenoma shares some morphologic features with FNH and, in fact, the former was previously termed "telangiectatic FNH" owing to the presence of nodules of hepatocytes separated by short fibrous septa (Fig. 1.23). Telangiectatic hepatocellular adenomas usually lack a central fibrous scar and their septa contain telangiectatic blood vessels, rather than proliferating bile ductules.

References

1. Cabibbo G, Craxi A. Needle track seeding following percutaneous procedures for hepatocellular carcinoma. World J Hepatol. 2009;31(1):62–6.
2. Liu C, Frilling A, Dereskewitz C, et al. Tumor seeding after fine needle aspiration biopsy and percutaneous radiofrequency thermal ablation of hepatocellular carcinoma. Dig Surg. 2003;20:460–3.
3. Chang S, Kim SH, Lim HK, et al. Needle tract implantation after percutaneous interventional procedures in hepatocellular carcinomas: lessons learned from a 10-year experience. Korean J Radiol. 2008;9(3):268–74.
4. Silva MA, Hegab B, Hyde C, Guo G, Buckels JA, Mirza DF. Needle track seeding following biopsy of liver lesions in the diagnosis of hepatocellular cancer: a systematic review and meta-analysis. Gut. 2008;57(11):1592–6.
5. Cha CH, Saif MW, Yamane BH, Weber SM. Hepatocellular carcinoma: current management. Curr Probl Surg. 2010;47(1):10–67.
6. Jemal A, Siegel R, Ward E, Hao Y, Xu J, Thun MJ. Cancer statistics 2009. CA Cancer J Clin. 2009;59(4):225–49.
7. El-Serag H, Mason AC, Key C. Trends in survival of patients with hepatocellular carcinoma between 1977 and 1996 in the United States. Hepatology. 2001;33(1):62–5.
8. El-Serag H. Epidemiology of hepatocellular carcinoma in USA. Hepatology. 2007;37 Suppl 2:S88–94.
9. Tsim NC, Frampton AE, Habib NA, Jiao LR. Surgical treatment for liver cancer. World J Gastroenterol. 2010;16(8):927–33.
10. Mazzaferro V, Regalia E, Doci R, et al. Liver transplantation for the treatment of small hepatocellular carcinomas in patients with cirrhosis. New Engl J Med. 1996;334:693–700.
11. Grazioli L, Federle MP, Ichikawa T, et al. Liver adenomatosis: clinical, histopathologic, and imaging findings in 15 patients. Radiology. 2000;216:395–402.
12. Foster JH, Donohue TA, Berman MM. Familial liver-cell adenomas and diabetes mellitus. N Engl J Med. 1978;299:239–41.

13. Labrune P, Trioche P, Duvaltier I, et al. Hepatocellular adenomas in glycogen storage disease type I and III: a series of 43 patients and review of the literature. J Pediatr Gastroenterol Nutr. 1997;24:276–9.
14. Cherqui D, Rahmouni A, Charlotte F, et al. Management of focal nodular hyperplasia and hepatocellular adenoma in young women: a series of 41 patients with clinical, radiological, and pathological correlations. Hepatology. 1995;22(6):1674–81.

Chapter 2
Intraoperative Evaluation of Hepatic Biliary Lesions

INTRODUCTION

Most hepatic biliary lesions are benign and incidentally discovered during procedures unrelated to the liver. Benign bile duct proliferations are gray–white subcapsular nodules that are often multiple, so it is not surprising that their detection results in more liver frozen sections than any other finding. In contrast, a diagnosis of intrahepatic cholangiocarcinoma is almost always known prior to surgery. Thus, diagnostic frozen sections are rarely performed. Cholangiocarcinomas that involve the liver occur either in the proximal extrahepatic bile ducts and directly extend into the liver (hilar cholangiocarcinoma or Klatskin tumor) or they arise from the intrahepatic biliary tree. Intrahepatic cholangiocarcinomas are subclassified in two broad groups based on their anatomic location in the porta hepatis and/or large ramifying ducts (central cholangiocarcinoma) or smaller ducts (peripheral cholangiocarcinoma). Intraoperative consultations for cholangiocarcinoma are usually limited to bile duct margin evaluation on tumors that involve the perihilar region, although surgeons may request evaluation of parenchymal margins for peripheral cholangiocarcinomas. In the former situation, frozen sections are obtained from the main hepatic resection specimen or separately submitted segments of extrahepatic bile duct. The purpose of this chapter is to discuss the following: (1) the histologic features of benign bile duct lesions, (2) criteria that aid their distinction from carcinoma, and (3) issues related to margins of resection for malignant biliary-type tumors that involve the liver. Extrahepatic biliary neoplasia is discussed in further detail in Chapter 6.

21

R.K. Yantiss (ed.), *Frozen Section Library: Liver, Extrahepatic Biliary Tree and Gallbladder*, Frozen Section Library, DOI 10.1007/978-1-4614-0043-1_2,
© Springer Science+Business Media, LLC 2011

BENIGN BILE DUCT LESIONS OF LIVER

Bile duct hamartomas (von Meyenberg complexes) and bile duct adenomas (biliary adenomas) are common, incidentally discovered lesions that generally escape preoperative detection because they are too small to be seen radiographically. Both types of lesion occur as solitary, or multiple, white nodules that span only a few millimeters and are more numerous under the capsule (Fig. 2.1). Their multifocal nature raises concern for possible metastatic disease and they are frequently submitted for intraoperative evaluation. In fact, they represent the most common indication for frozen section evaluation of the liver and one of the most challenging problems encountered in the frozen section laboratory [1, 2]. The distinguishing features of benign ductal lesions and metastatic adenocarcinoma are summarized in Table 2.1.

Bile Duct Hamartoma (von Meyenberg Complex)

Bile duct hamartomas are well-circumscribed aggregates of biliary ductules embedded in a near-equal amount of hyalinized stroma (Fig. 2.2). These ductules are variably cystic and lined by flattened, or cuboidal, epithelium without cytologic atypia. Some bile duct hamartomas contain inspissated bile, but this finding is inconsistently present (Figs. 2.3 and 2.4). Multiple bile duct hamartomas are distributed along the portal tracts, reflecting their

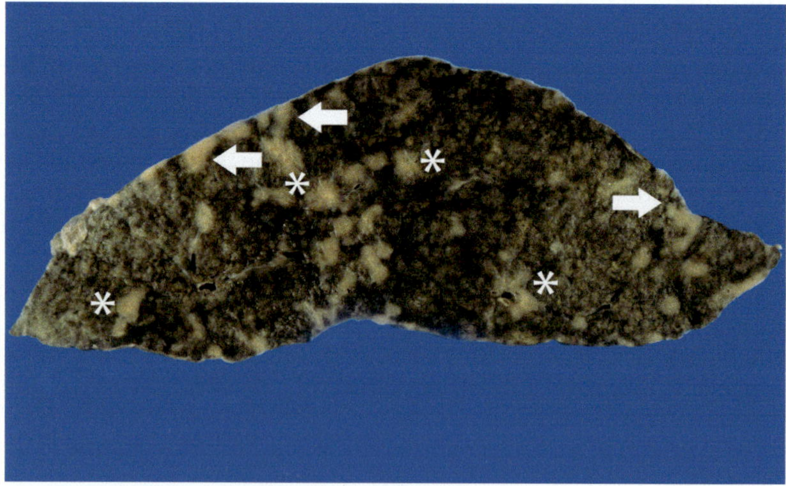

Fig. 2.1 Multiple von Meyenberg complexes (bile duct hamartomas) are present under the capsule (*arrows*) and adjacent to portal tracts (*asterisks*).

TABLE 2.1 Features that distinguish between benign bile duct proliferations and metastatic adenocarcinoma.

Feature	Bile duct hamartoma	Bile duct adenoma	Metastatic adenocarcinoma
Anatomic location	Subcapsular	Subcapsular	Variable
Size	<1 cm	<1 cm	Variable
Tumor centricity	Solitary or multiple	Solitary or multiple	Usually multiple
Quality of stroma	Densely collagenous	Cellular	Desmoplastic
Appearance	Circumscribed	Circumscribed	Ill-defined
Intralesional portal tracts	Common	Common	Present at lesional edge
Organization of epithelium	Uniformly-spaced, variably dilated tubules	Uniformly-spaced, small round tubules	Irregular aggregates of variably sized glands
Luminal mucin	Absent	May be present	Present
Bile	May be present	Absent	Absent
Cytologic atypia	Absent	Minimal	Present
Mitoses	Absent	Absent	Present

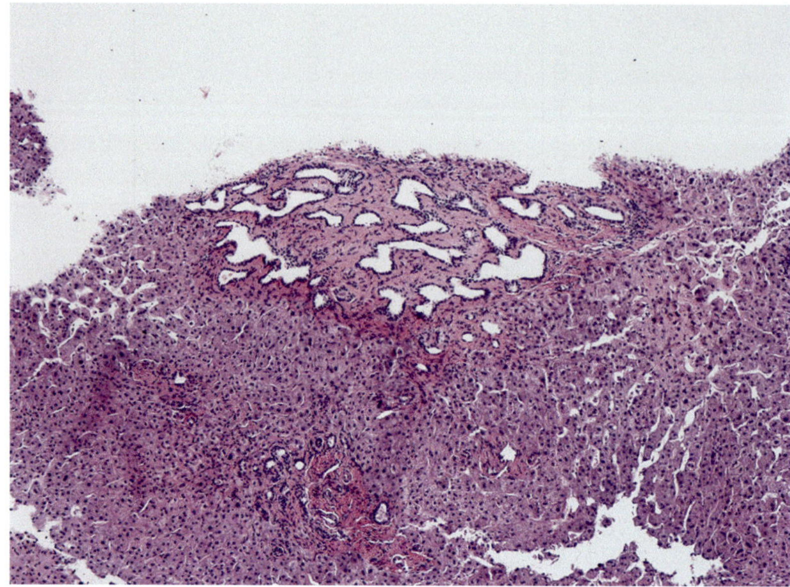

FIG. 2.2 Bile duct hamartomas are well-circumscribed proliferations of dilated tubules associated with collagenous stroma.

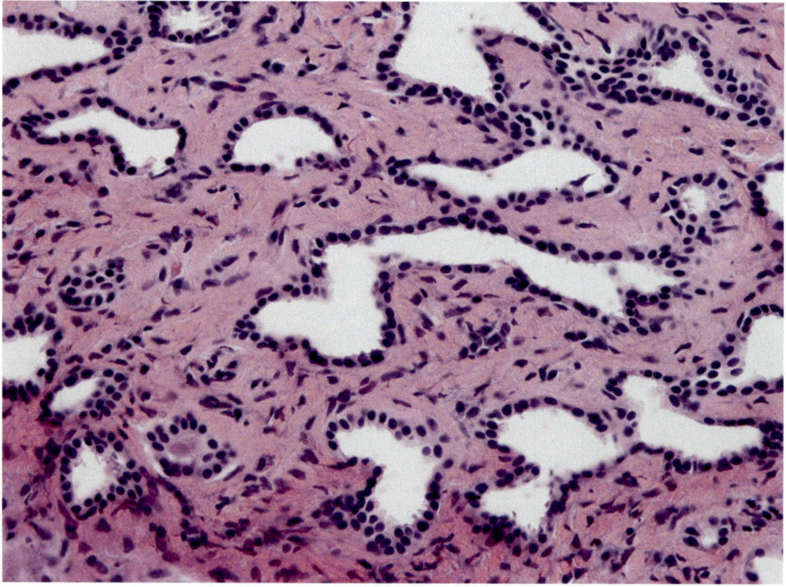

FIG. 2.3 The tubules of a bile duct hamartoma are lined by cuboidal, or flattened, epithelial cells that lack cytologic atypia. The stroma is dense, paucicellular, and eosinophilic.

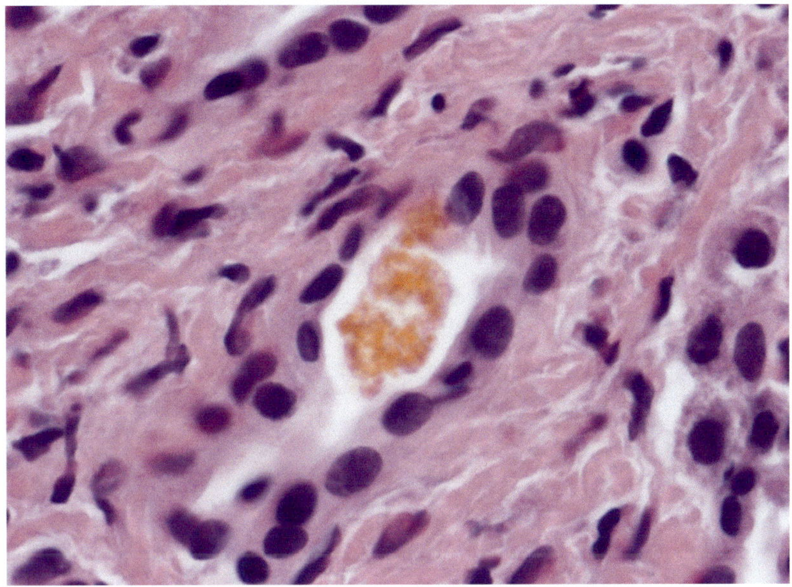

Fɪɢ. 2.4 Inspissated bile is present within the tubules of a bile duct hamartoma.

origin from malformations at the interface between limiting plate hepatocytes and the portal tracts (Fig. 2.5). Most bile duct hamartomas are readily distinguished from metastatic adenocarcinoma at low magnification. Bile duct hamartomas are round aggregates of ductules embedded in dense paucicellular collagen, whereas carcinoma deposits are ill-defined, expansile nodules composed of irregularly spaced glands and single cells enmeshed in desmoplastic stroma (Fig. 2.6). Carcinomatous glands are haphazardly arranged and angulated with highly atypical cells (Fig. 2.7).

Bile Duct Adenoma (Biliary Adenoma)

Bile duct adenomas are well-circumscribed proliferations of small tubules and stroma that are morphologically distinct from bile duct hamartomas (Fig. 2.8). They contain densely packed, proliferating ductules enmeshed within compact, cellular stroma (Fig. 2.9). These ductules are lined by plump, cuboidal epithelial cells with abundant faintly eosinophilic cytoplasm and display mild, if any, cytologic atypia (Fig. 2.10). Bile duct adenomas do not contain bile. Their recognition is quite problematic in some cases because the cellular stroma may simulate desmoplasia and the dense proliferation

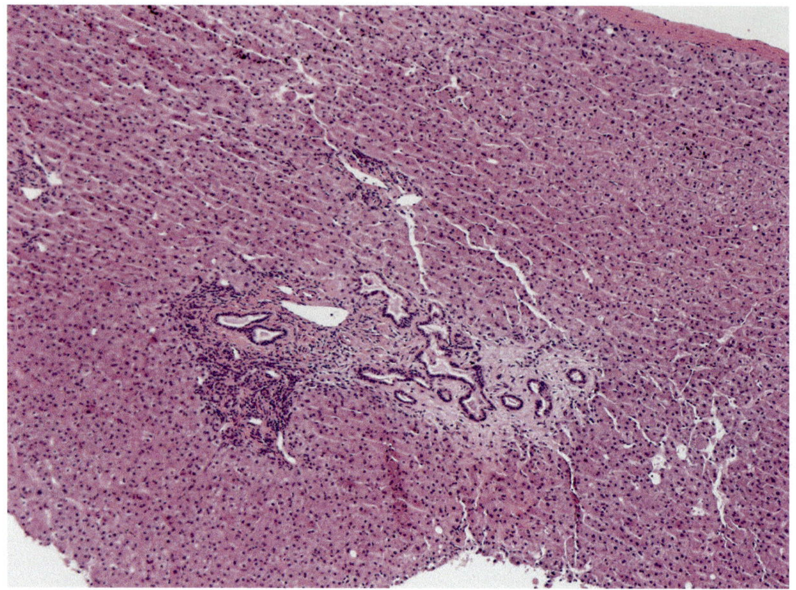

FIG. 2.5 Bile duct hamartomas occur along portal tracts and are often multiple.

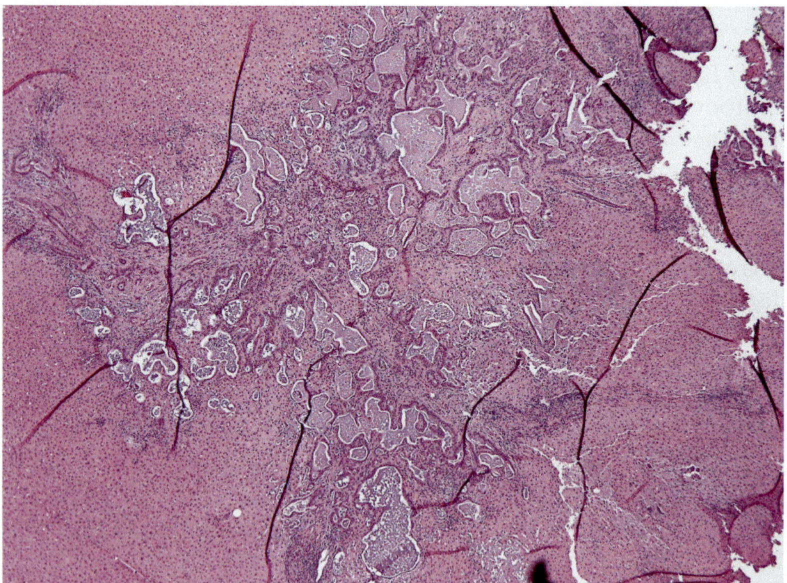

FIG. 2.6 Metastatic pancreatic ductal adenocarcinoma is an ill-defined, expansile nodule composed of irregularly spaced glands that are variably dilated and contain mucin.

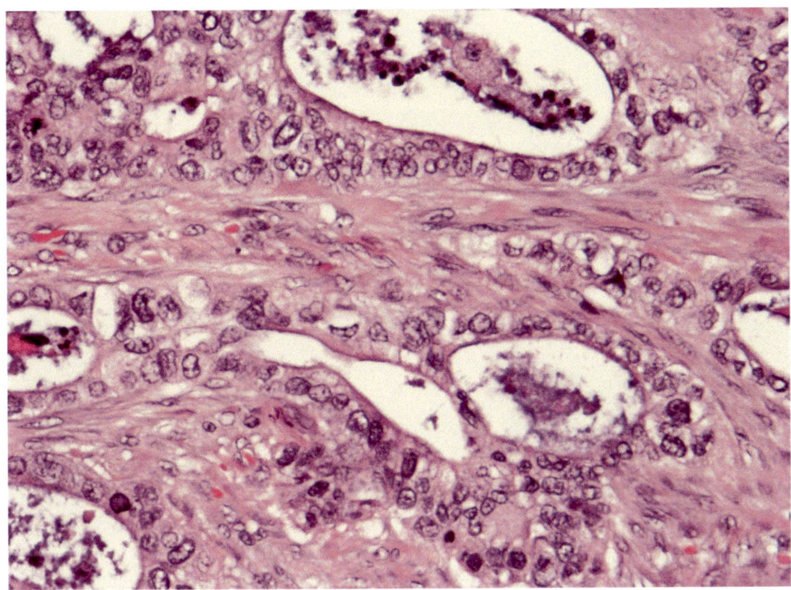

FIG. 2.7 The infiltrative glands of metastatic pancreatic ductal adenocarcinoma are embedded in desmoplastic stroma. They are variable in size and shape and contain epithelial cells with severe cytologic atypia.

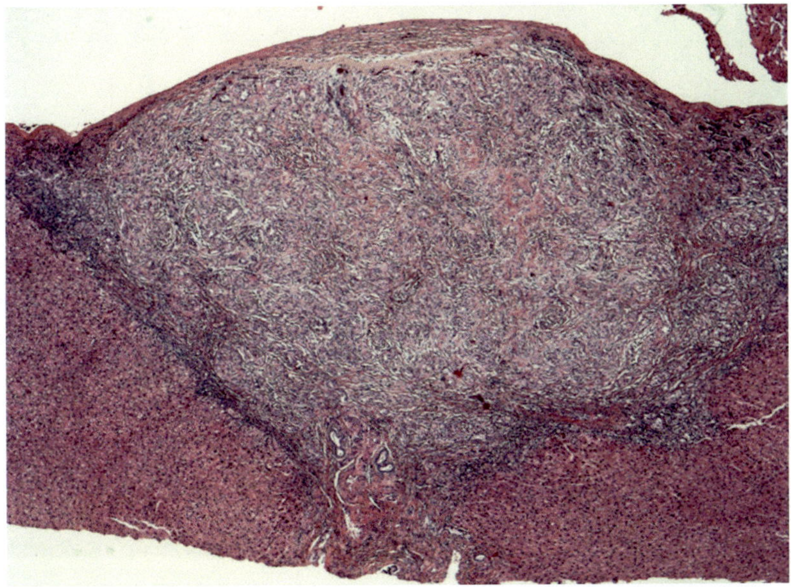

FIG. 2.8 Bile duct adenomas are well-circumscribed subcapsular proliferative lesions that contain numerous glands and stroma.

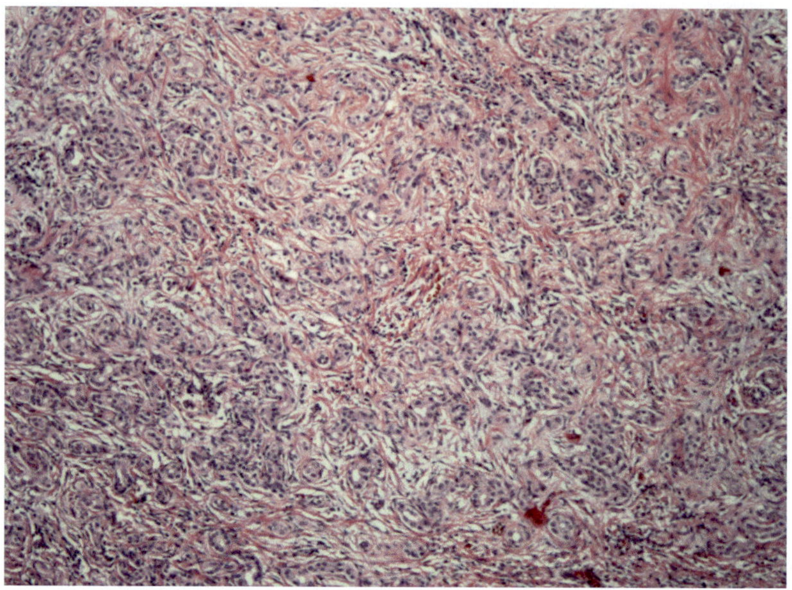

FIG. 2.9 The glands of a bile duct adenoma are densely-packed and surrounded by cellular stroma.

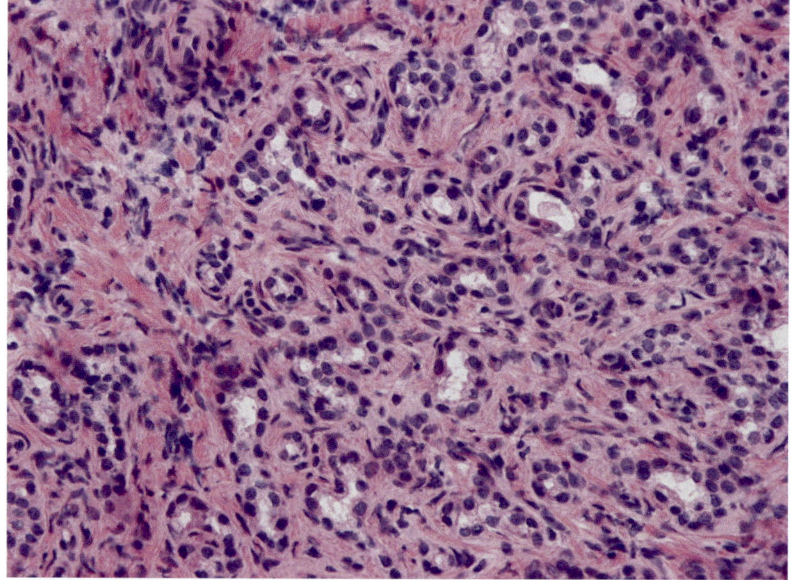

FIG. 2.10 Bile duct adenomas contain proliferating tubules lined by cuboidal cells with faintly eosinophilic cytoplasm and round nuclei. The stroma contains inflammatory cells, but is not desmoplastic.

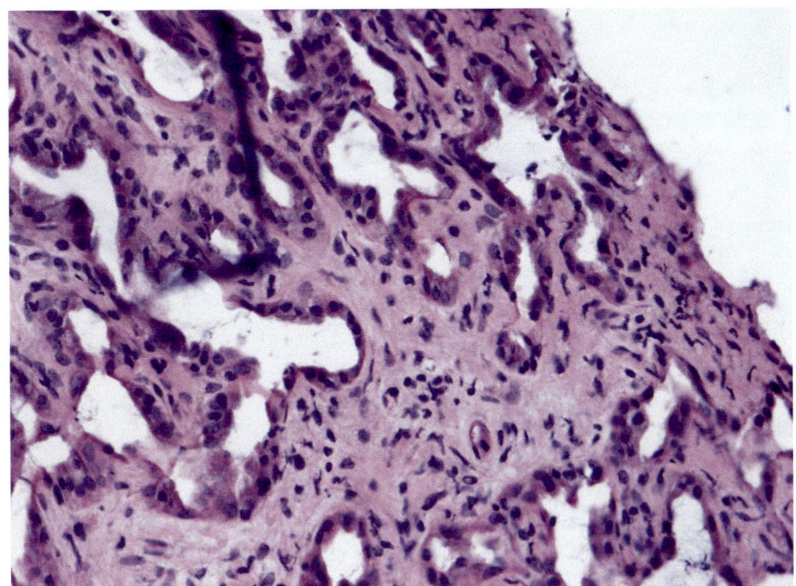

FIG. 2.11   Frozen section artifact may enhance cytologic atypia in bile duct adenomas.

of slightly atypical ducts may be mistaken for adenocarcinoma, particularly when the degree of cytologic atypia is enhanced by frozen section artifact (Fig. 2.11). This problem is compounded when bile duct adenomas contain mucin, since this finding has been considered a feature of adenocarcinoma (Fig. 2.12). Other criteria that aid the distinction between bile duct adenoma and adenocarcinoma include the well-circumscribed appearance of the former, the nature of its stroma, and presence of only mild cytologic atypia in these lesions.

Inflammatory Changes in Preexisting Bile Ducts

Patients with chronic ascending cholangitis develop persistent localized ductal dilatation in combination with hepatic scarring that may simulate the appearance of either primary or metastatic adenocarcinoma (Fig. 2.13). Carcinomas of the pancreatic head, distal bile duct, and/or ampulla may cause bile duct obstruction that produces ductular reactions in the liver that grow large enough to be identified during surgery. Large duct obstruction typically results in a bile ductular proliferation in the portal tracts with periportal edema and fibrosis. The ductules are variably dilated

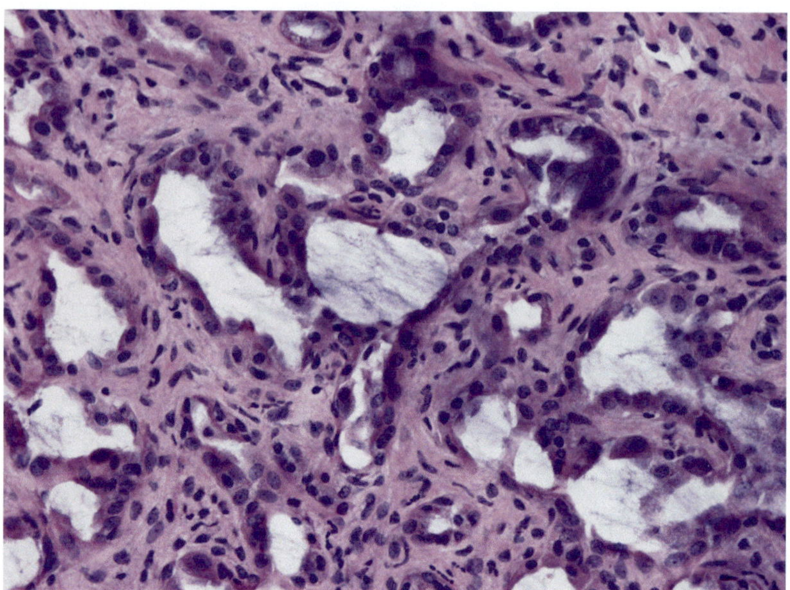

Fig. 2.12 Some bile duct adenomas contain mucin, which should not be interpreted as a diagnostic feature of metastatic adenocarcinoma.

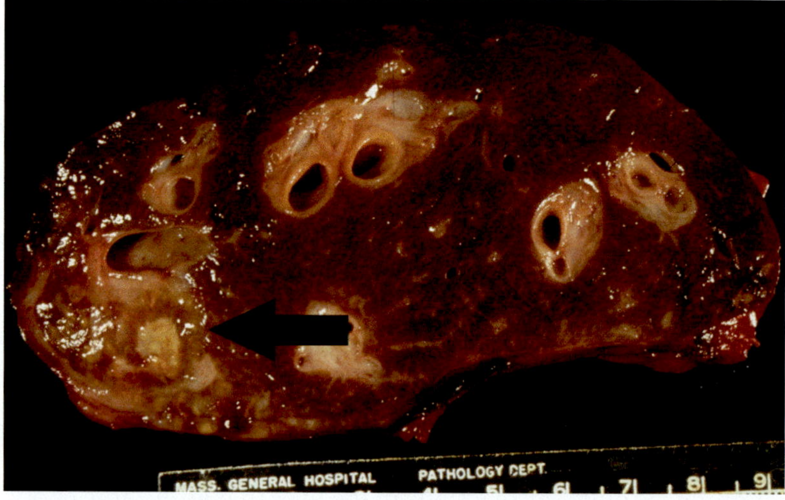

Fig. 2.13 Chronic ascending cholangitis causes dilatation of bile ducts with periportal fibrosis. Localized organizing abscesses in the parenchyma form an ill-defined mass (*arrow*).

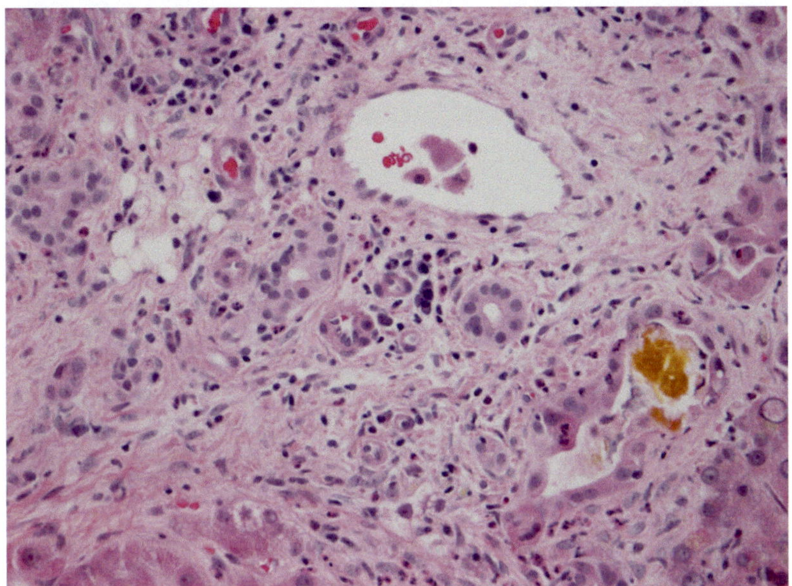

FIG. 2.14 Large duct obstruction causes bile ductular proliferation in portal tracts. The ducts are variable in size and some contain bile.

and show mild cytologic atypia with bile plugs and neutrophils, but they do not infiltrate adjacent parenchyma (Fig. 2.14). Long-standing obstruction may lead to extensive ductular proliferation in combination with inflammatory stroma that forms a mass. These ductules can simulate adenocarcinoma, especially when entrapped ductules appear angulated or compressed (Figs. 2.15 and 2.16).

Distinction Between Benign and Malignant Glandular Lesions in the Liver

Metastatic adenocarcinomas of the pancreaticobiliary tree, stomach, esophagus, and gastroesophageal junction are close mimics of benign bile duct proliferations, especially bile duct adenomas. Helpful distinguishing features include the well-circumscribed nature of benign lesions and their near-complete lack of cytologic atypia (Table 2.1). Some hepatic nodules may not be classifiable as benign or malignant based upon frozen section analysis alone. In this situation, it is best to communicate concerns to the surgeon and defer final classification to permanent sections. An incorrect diagnosis of benignancy will result in continuation of surgery and resection of the primary tumor, whereas a diagnosis of metastatic

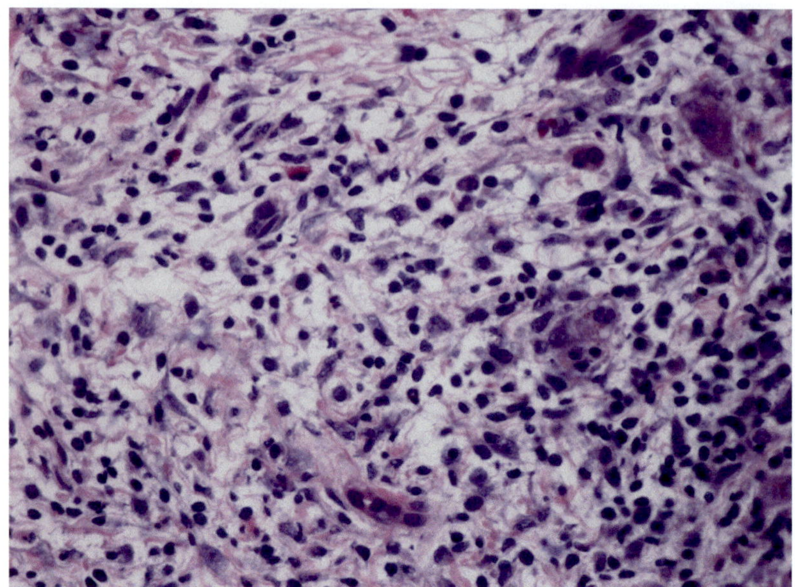

Fig. 2.15 Large duct obstruction may produce nodules of proliferating ductules associated with inflammation and loose inflammatory stroma.

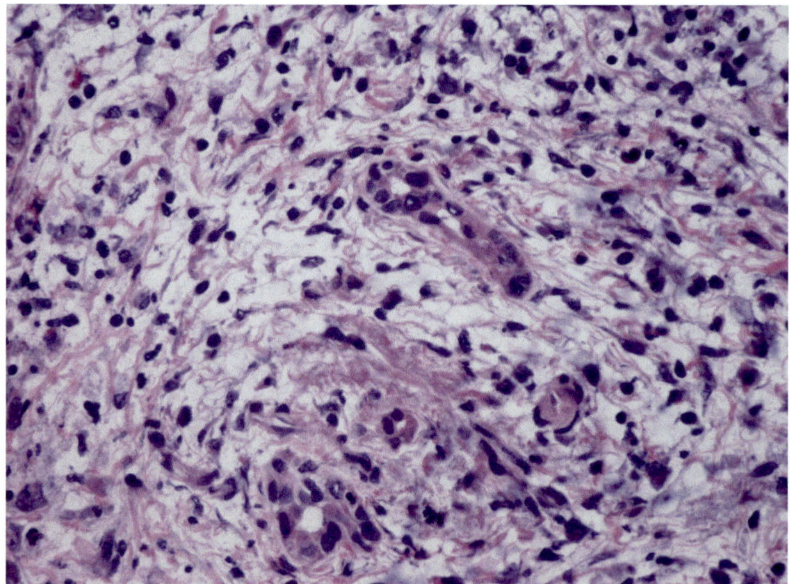

Fig. 2.16 This patient had an obstructing pancreatic adenocarcinoma and a small hepatic nodule that was intraoperatively assessed during pancreatectomy. Angulated proliferating bile ducts in myxoid stroma mimic metastatic carcinoma. The frozen section interpretation was further hampered by knowledge that the patient had received neoadjuvant chemotherapy, which might be expected to induce fibrosis around metastatic carcinoma (same case as Fig. 2.15).

TABLE 2.2 Immunohistochemical stains that distinguish bile duct adenoma from metastatic carcinoma.

Immunohistochemical stain	Bile duct adenoma	Metastatic adenocarcinoma
p53	Negative	Positive
TAG-72	Negative	Positive
mCEA	Negative	Positive
Mesothelin	Negative	Positive
BCL2	Negative	Positive
IMP3	Negative	Positive
CA125	Negative	Positive
AMACR	Negative	Positive
DPC4	Positive	Negative
Ki67	<35% staining of lesional nuclei	>35% staining of lesional nuclei

Based on data from: Hornick et al. [3]; Tan et al. [15]

carcinoma will halt the procedure. We have, on rare occasion, asked the surgeon to delay a procedure to evaluate permanent sections and ensure a correct diagnosis. Immunohistochemical stains may also be used to facilitate the distinction between benign ductular proliferations and metastatic adenocarcinoma (Table 2.2) [3].

Mucinous Cystadenoma (Hepatobiliary Cystadenoma)

Mucinous cystadenoma of the liver was first described in association with pancreatic mucinous cystic neoplasms [4]. These tumors are more common among women and are unilocular, or multilocular, cysts with internal septations. Potentially life-threatening complications such as bleeding or perforation due to erosion into adjacent structures may occur [5]. Hepatic mucinous cystadenomas contain epithelial cells that resemble endocervical epithelium and show a spectrum of cytologic atypia, ranging from low- to high-grade dysplasia. Rare tumors precede invasive carcinoma. Mucinous cystadenomas in women typically contain dense "ovarian-type stroma," whereas those that arise in men lack this feature (Fig. 2.17) [6]. Complete surgical removal is the treatment of choice in patients with symptomatic disease, radiographic features suspicious for malignancy, and high-grade epithelial cell dysplasia in material obtained by fine needle aspiration. Intraoperative consultations may be obtained to assess the adequacy of surgical

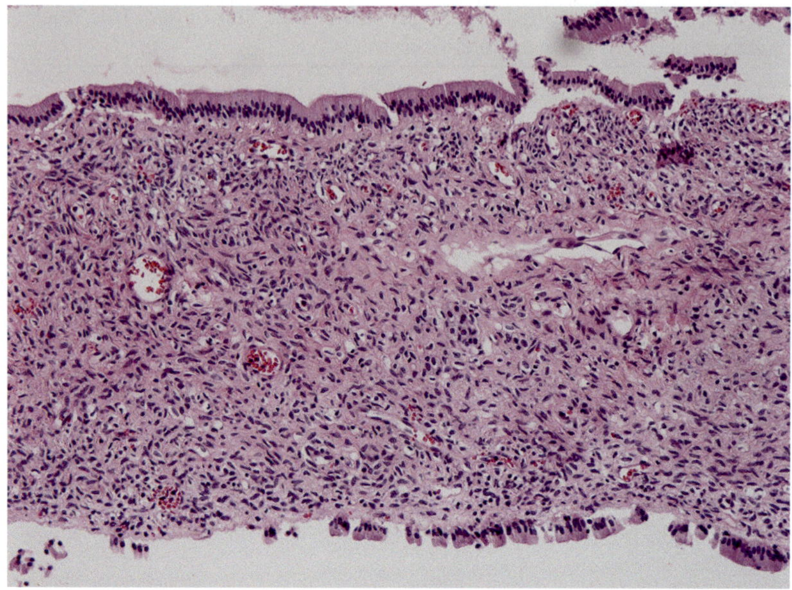

Fɪɢ. 2.17 Mucinous cystadenomas contain epithelium that resembles endocervical cells overlying dense "ovarian-type stroma." This tumor shows only low-grade dysplasia in lesional epithelium.

resection or to make a primary diagnosis in those cases that have not been previously evaluated by cytology [7].

MALIGNANT BILE DUCT LESIONS OF THE LIVER

Cholangiocarcinomas are malignant epithelial tumors derived from the intrahepatic and/or extrahepatic bile ducts. These aggressive neoplasms are classified based upon their anatomic location. Those that develop within the liver are intrahepatic cholangiocarcinomas and are classified as central and peripheral types. Extrahepatic cholangiocarcinomas that arise at the bifurcation of right and left hepatic ducts are subclassified as proximal (hilar) cholangiocarcinomas, and distal cholangiocarcinomas occur distal to the bifurcation. Frozen section analysis of bile duct margin is commonly performed to guide the extent of resection for cholangiocarcinomas of the perihilar region, including both extrahepatic tumors that invade the liver (hilar cholangiocarcinoma or Klatskin tumor) and those that develop in the porta hepatis (intrahepatic central cholangiocarcinoma). Pathologists may be asked to perform frozen sections on bile duct margins present in hepatic resection specimens or separately submitted segments of extrahepatic bile duct distal to the tumor. Extrahepatic cholangiocarcinomas are discussed in detail in Chapter 6.

The reported risk factors for, and natural history of, intrahepatic cholangiocarcinoma mostly reflect the features of central tumors, which are much more common than peripheral lesions. Risk factors for development of cholangiocarcinoma include primary sclerosing cholangitis, hepatolithiasis, and parasitic infestation of the biliary tree by *Opisthorchis viverrini* and *Clonorchis sinensis* [8]. These liver flukes are endemic to parts of southeast and eastern Asia and account for the striking geographic distribution of intrahepatic cholangiocarcinoma [9]. The incidence of intrahepatic cholangiocarcinoma in the United States has been steadily increasing since the 1970s for unclear reasons, although it is notable that this rise parallels a concurrent increase in HCV infection rates [8]. Central cholangiocarcinoma is associated with a poor prognosis, and surgical resection is the only curative therapy since adjuvant therapy is of limited efficacy in disease management. Unfortunately, many patients have advanced tumors at clinical presentation or extensive hepatic fibrosis and insufficient hepatic reserves to undergo liver resection [10, 11]. Liver transplantation is a consideration in latter situation, provided patients have localized tumors, although approximately 50% of cholangiocarcinomas recur in the graft liver [11].

Central Cholangiocarcinoma

Central cholangiocarcinomas are ill-defined, gritty, gray–white masses that track along the central portal structures in proximity to the bile duct and or portal vein margins (Fig. 2.18). Most do not develop in patients with cirrhosis (Fig. 2.19). Often, the ligated bile duct, artery, and vein are not readily identifiable on hepatic resection specimens and, thus, must be clearly indicated by the surgeon. Frozen sections are routinely obtained on bile duct margins to confirm adequate tumor clearance and an absence of dysplasia, which may appear as a mucosal irregularity in the bile duct (Figs. 2.20 and 2.21). Sections of vascular and bile duct margins are generally taken *en face*, although one may argue that perpendicular sections provide a more accurate estimate of tumor clearance than *en face* margins. Indeed, submillimeter assessment of margins is probably an academic exercise. Patients with narrow (<1 mm), but negative, bile duct resection margins have recurrence rates similar to those of patients with microscopically positive margins (Fig. 2.22) [12, 13].

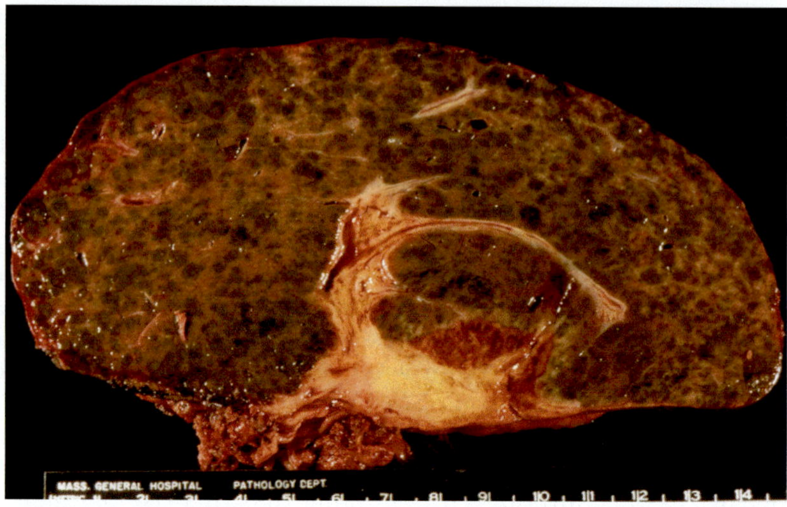

FIG. 2.18 This central cholangiocarcinomas is a firm yellow–white tumor at the hilum. It is associated with bile staining of the liver due to obstruction.

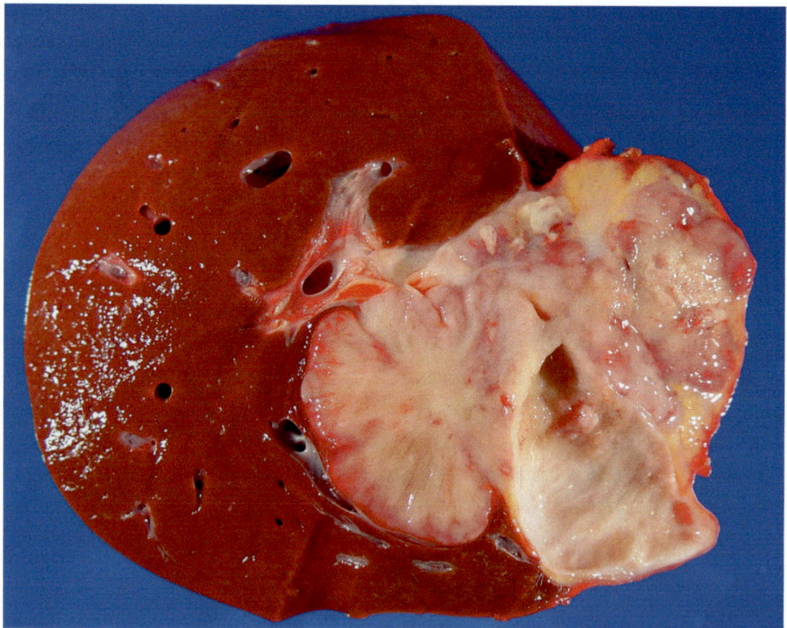

FIG. 2.19 This central cholangiocarcinoma encases the hilar structures. The background liver is essentially normal.

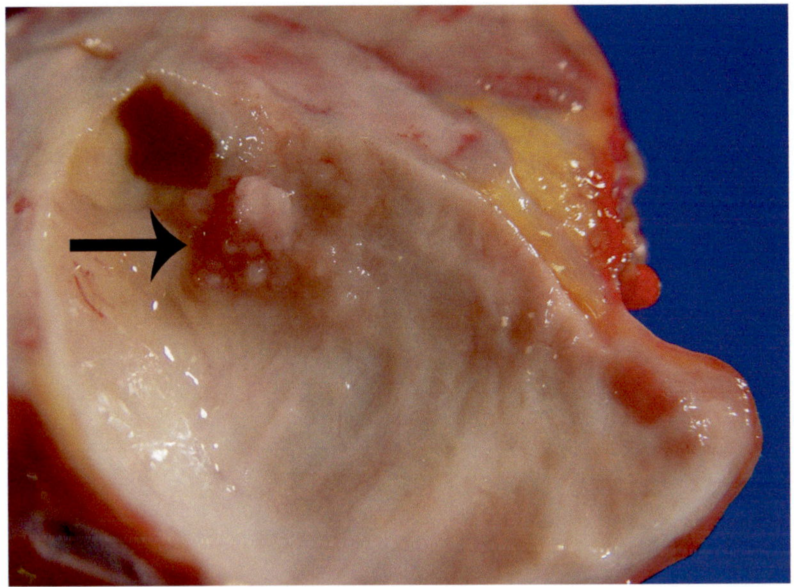

FIG. 2.20 Polypoid lesions in the duct raise concern for neoplasia (*arrow*) and, prompt frozen section evaluation of the bile duct resection margin (same case as Fig. 2.19).

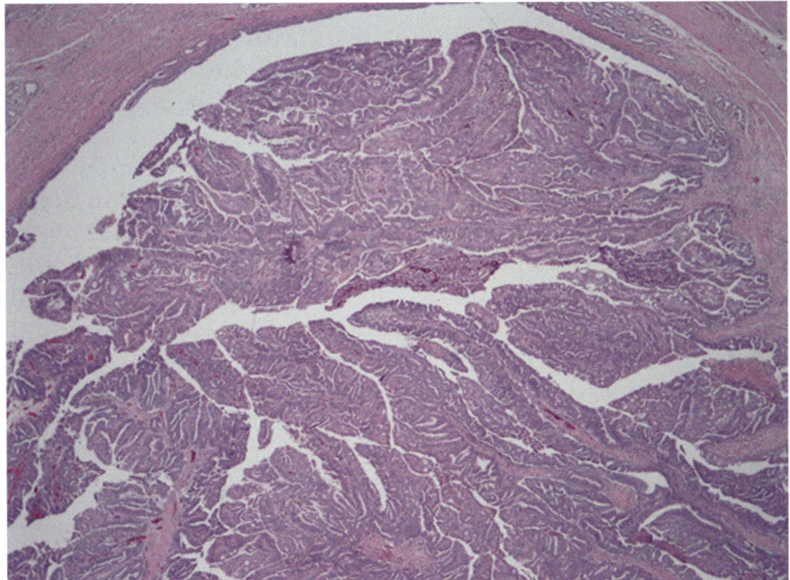

FIG. 2.21 Frozen section of the polypoid lesion (same case as Fig. 2.20) reveals a complex papillary proliferation of dysplastic epithelium.

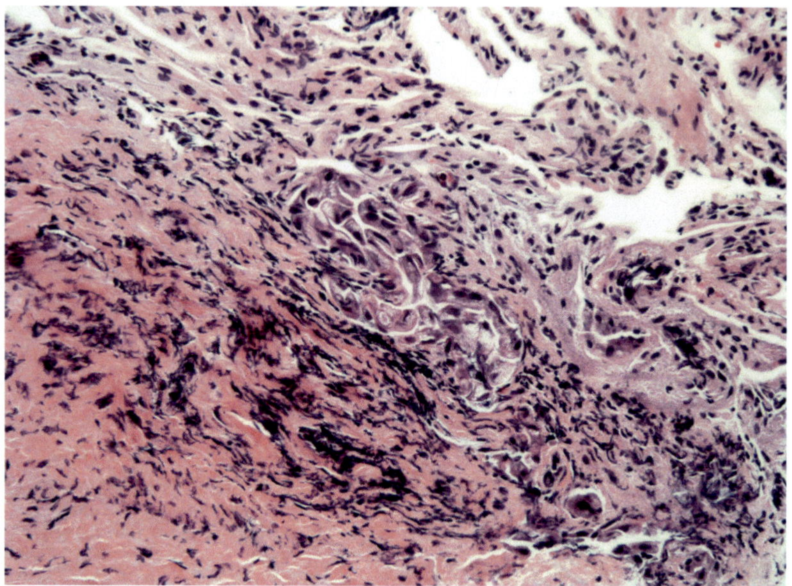

FIG. 2.22 Malignant glands enmeshed in desmoplastic stroma are present at the resection margin of this cholangiocarcinoma.

Outcomes are superior among patients with widely negative bile duct margins, such as those individuals with negative margins on both hepatic resection specimens and separately submitted bile duct segments [14].

Central and hilar cholangiocarcinomas contain overtly malignant, infiltrating glands and single cells enmeshed within desmoplastic stroma, similar to pancreatic ductal adenocarcinomas (Fig. 2.23). The diagnosis is generally straightforward when evaluating the primary tumor, but assessing bile duct margins is challenging. Invasive cholangiocarcinomas usually invade the bile duct wall, but spare the overlying mucosa (Fig. 2.24). Initial evaluation of bile duct margins is best achieved at low magnification, to appreciate the lobular architecture of benign periductal glands and distinguish them from infiltrating adenocarcinoma (Fig. 2.25). Periductal glands of the biliary mucosa show some degree of atypia due to either frozen section artifact or prior placement of a biliary stent (Figs. 2.26 and 2.27). Features suggesting a benign diagnosis include a rounded lobular architecture and mild atypia. This topic is discussed in further detail in Chapter 6.

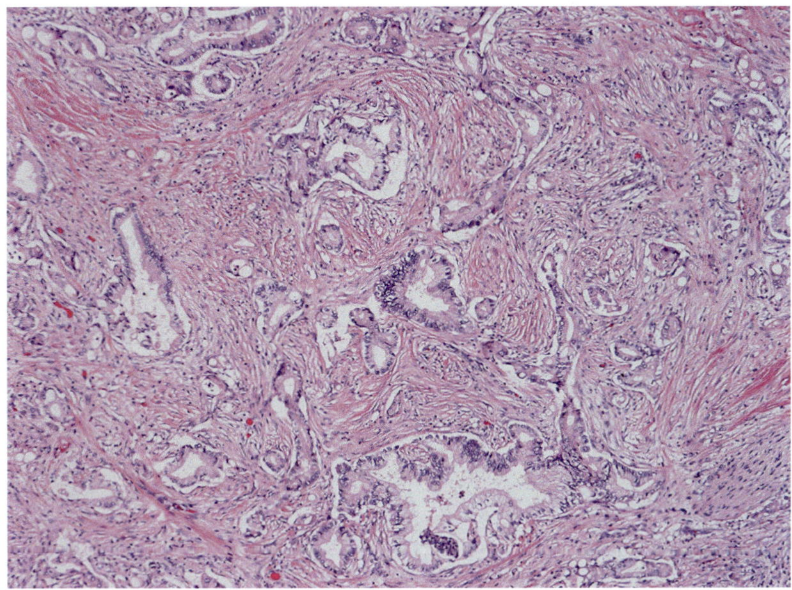

FIG. 2.23   Central cholangiocarcinomas contain irregularly spaced dilated glands associated with abundant desmoplastic stroma, similar to pancreatic ductal adenocarcinoma.

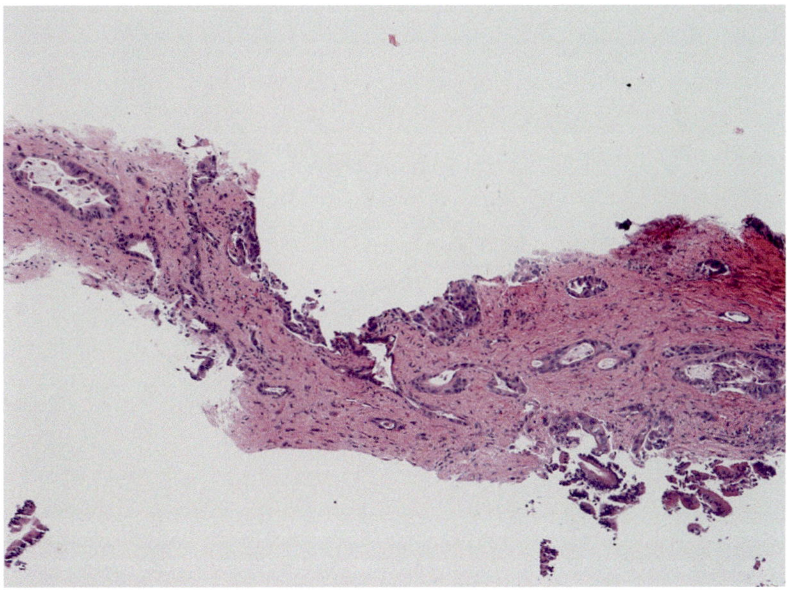

FIG. 2.24   The epithelium of this bile duct is partially denuded and the wall of the duct is infiltrated by cholangiocarcinoma.

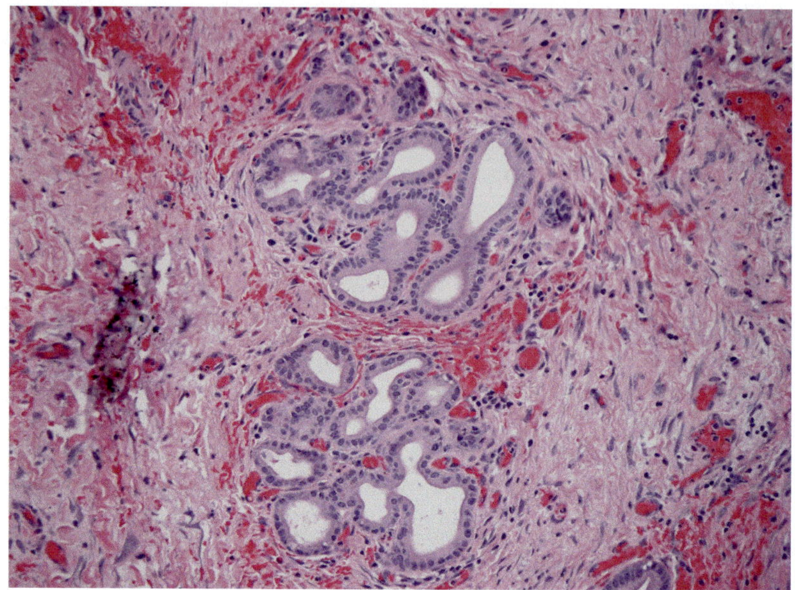

FIG. 2.25 Benign periductal glands are arranged in lobules and contain cells with round, regular, basally located nuclei and faintly eosinophilic cytoplasm.

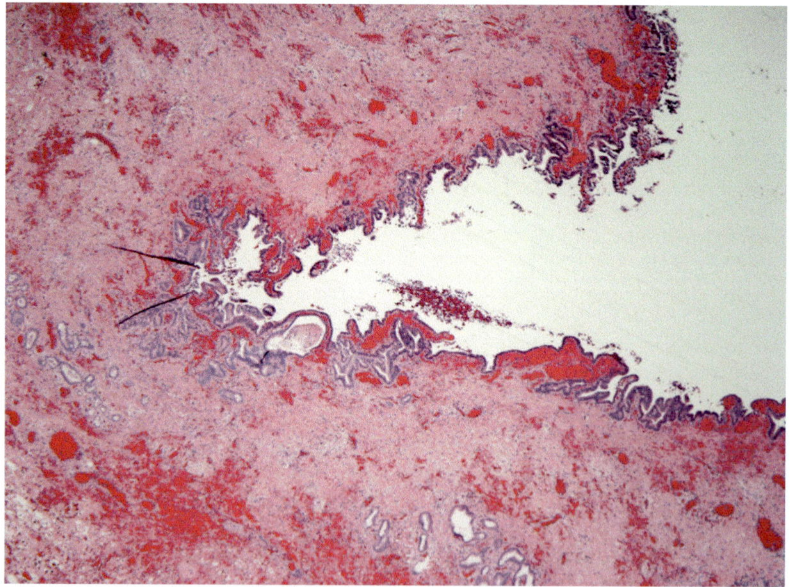

FIG. 2.26 The epithelium of a previously stented bile duct is proliferative and displays a slightly papillary architecture.

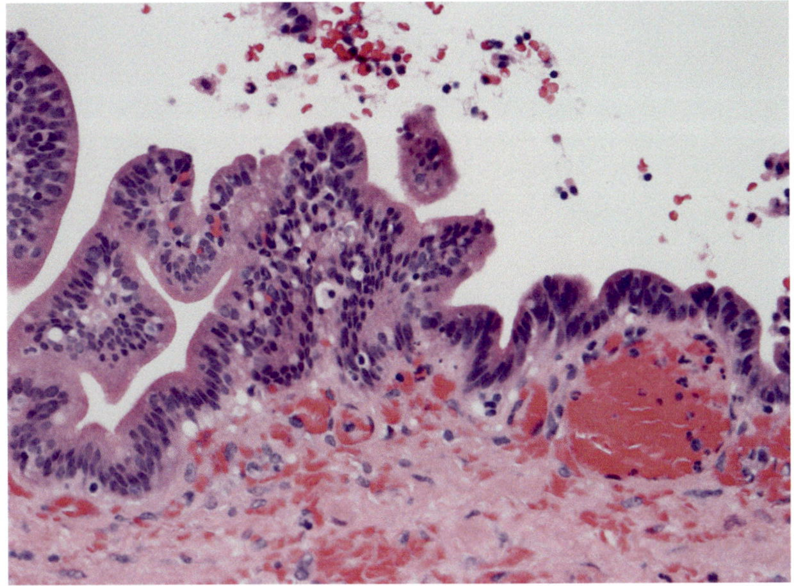

FIG. 2.27   This previously stented bile duct margin contains epithelial cells with mildly enlarged, basally oriented nuclei suggesting that the cytologic atypia is reactive (same case as Fig. 2.26).

Peripheral Cholangiocarcinoma

Peripheral cholangiocarcinomas are pale, relatively well-circumscribed, fleshy masses that occur distant from the hilum (Fig. 2.28). Most are resected *via* partial hepatectomy, so the most important margin is the hepatic parenchymal margin, which is inked and sectioned to demonstrate its relationship to the tumor (Figs. 2.28 and 2.29). Peripheral cholangiocarcinomas are morphologically distinct from central tumors, in that they are more cellular and composed of well-differentiated, neoplastic tubules with little intervening stroma (Fig. 2.30). The neoplastic cells are embedded in collagenous stroma that may be hyalinized (Fig. 2.31). Some tumors, particularly those in patients with underlying liver disease, have features of both adenocarcinoma and hepatocellular carcinoma (mixed hepatocellular/cholangiocarcinoma).

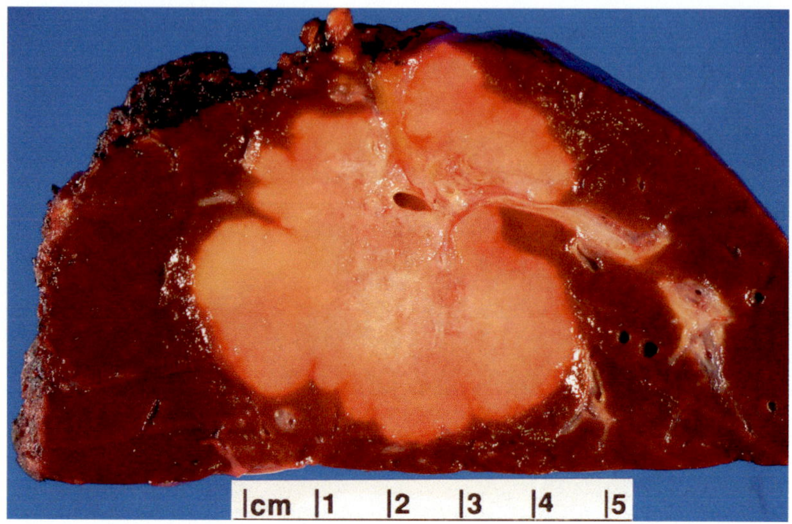

FIG. 2.28 Most peripheral cholangiocarcinomas are yellow–white solitary tumors with a scalloped edge. The background liver is usually normal.

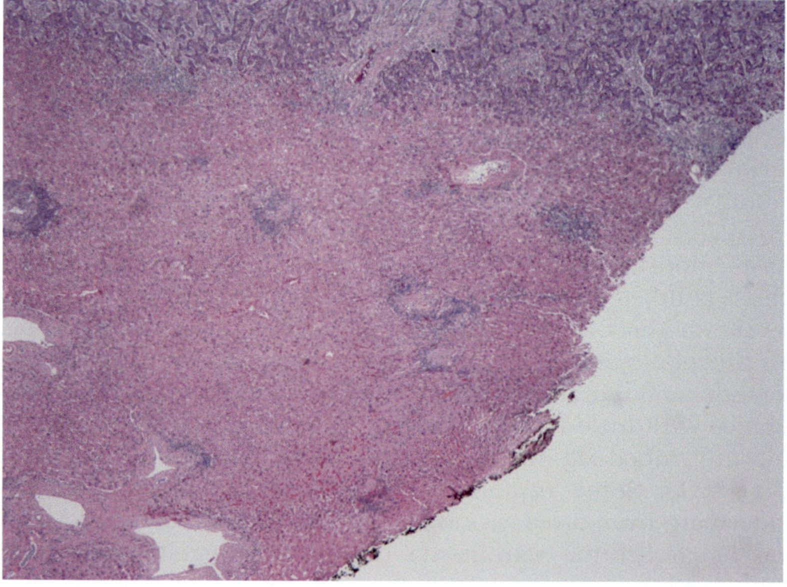

FIG. 2.29 This peripheral cholangiocarcinoma is 3 mm from the inked hepatic resection margin.

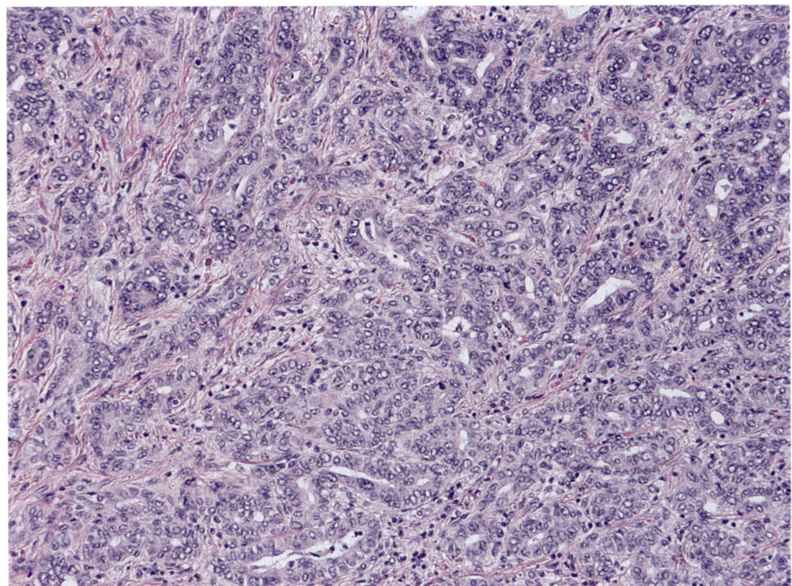

FIG. 2.30 Peripheral cholangiocarcinomas consist of well-differentiated tubules that may show minimal cytologic atypia.

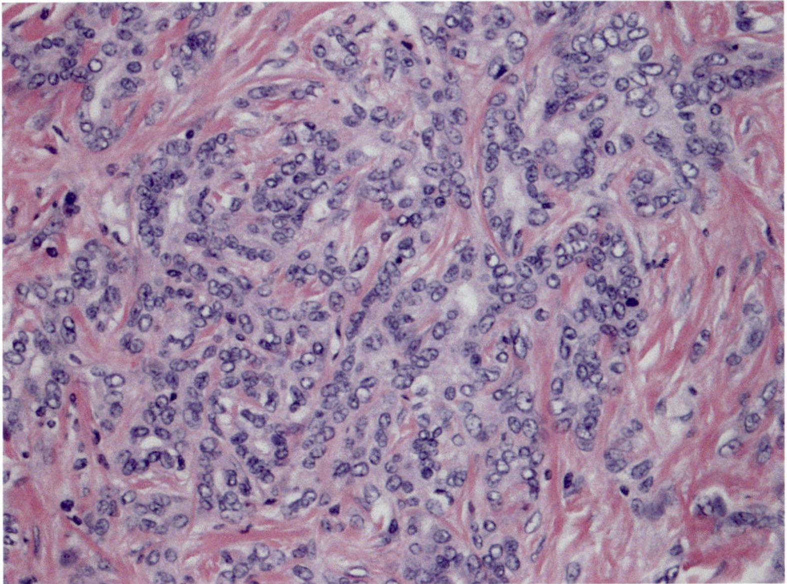

FIG. 2.31 The glands of peripheral cholangiocarcinoma are embedded in hyalinized or collagenous stroma that is less cellular than the desmoplatic stroma typical of central cholangiocarcinomas.

References

1. Guiu B, Guiu S, Loffroy R, Cercueil JP, Krause D. Multiple biliary hamartomas mimicking diffuse liver metastases. Dig Surg. 2009; 26(3):209.
2. Fritz S, Hackert T, Blaker H, et al. Multiple von Meyenberg complexes mimicking diffuse liver metastases from esophageal squamous cell carcinoma. World J Gastroenterol. 2006;12(26):4250–2.
3. Hornick JL, Lauwers GY, Odze RD. Immunohistochemistry can help distinguish metastatic pancreatic adenocarcinomas from bile duct adenomas and bile duct hamartomas of the liver. Am J Surg Pathol. 2005;29(3):381–9.
4. Brachet D, Mucci S, Desolneux G, et al. The simultaneous occurrence of mucinous cystadenomas in the liver and pancreas. Eur J Gastroenterol Hepatol. 2007;19(9):801–4.
5. Bacher H, Cerwenka H, Werkgartner G, et al. Primary biliary cystadenocarcinoma perforating the duodenum and left intrahepatic biliary tree-mimicking a hydatid cyst. Liver. 1999;19(1):39–41.
6. Devaney K, Goodman ZD, Ishak KG. Hepatobiliary cystadenoma and cystadenocarcinoma. A light microscopic and immunohistochemical study of 70 patients. Am J Surg. 1994;18(11):1078–91.
7. Iemoto Y, Kondo Y, Fukumachi S. Biliary cystadenocarcinoma with peritoneal carcinomatosis. Cancer. 1981;48(7):1664–7.
8. Patel T. Increasing incidence and mortality of primary intrahepatic cholangiocarcinoma in the United States. Hepatology. 2001;33(6): 1353–7.
9. Patel T. Worldwide trends in mortality from biliary tract malignancies. BMC Cancer. 2002;2:10. doi:10.1186/1471-2407-2-10.
10. Morise Z, Sugioka A, Tokoro T, et al. Surgery and chemotherapy for intrahepatic cholangiocarcinoma. World J Hepatol. 2010;2(2):58–64.
11. Rosen CB, Heimbach JK, Gores J. Surgery for cholangiocarcinoma: the role of liver transplantation. HPB. 2008;10(3):186–9.
12. Shingu Y, Ebata T, Nishio H, Igami T, Shimoyama Y, Nagino M. Clinical value of additional resection of a margin-positive proximal bile duct in hilar cholangiocarcinoma. Surgery. 2010;147(1):49–56.
13. Sasaki R, Takeda Y, Funato O, et al. Significance of ductal margin status in patients undergoing surgical resection for extrahepatic cholangiocarcinoma. World J Surg. 2007;31(9):1788–96.
14. Endo I, House MG, Klimstra DS, et al. Clinical significance of intraoperative bile duct margin assessment for hilar cholangiocarcinoma. Ann Surg Oncol. 2008;15(8):2104–12.
15. Tan G, Yilmaz A, DeYoung BR, Behling C, Lehman A, Frankel WL. Immunohistochemical analysis of biliary tract lesions. Appl Immunohistochem Mol Morphol. 2004;12(3):193–7.

Chapter 3
Metastases and Mimics of Metastatic Disease in the Liver

INTRODUCTION

Most malignant hepatic tumors are metastases, which outnumber hepatocellular carcinoma by 40:1 in Europe and North America [1]. Hepatic sinusoidal fenestrations and a rich vascular supply derived from branches of the portal vein and hepatic artery facilitate parenchymal invasion by malignant cells, so it is not surprising that the liver is a frequent site of metastasis, being second only to regional lymph nodes. Carcinomas of the tubular gut and pancreas show a propensity to metastasize to the liver. Nongastrointestinal malignancies that frequently disseminate to the liver include malignant melanoma and carcinomas of the lung and breast [2, 3]. Mesenchymal neoplasms, especially gastrointestinal stromal tumors (GISTs), and endocrine neoplasms of the pancreas, tubular gut, and lung also spread to the liver. Preoperative or intraoperative detection of hepatic metastases is important because it is often a contraindication to further surgery for the primary tumor, especially in patients with primary carcinomas of the esophagus, stomach, and pancreas. Radiographic studies usually provide accurate preoperative staging information for patients with extrahepatic malignancies, although surgeons may observe unsuspected abnormalities during exploratory laparotomy that warrant frozen section analysis.

Metastatic tumor deposits in the liver may be amenable to surgical excision in selected cases. Some patients with stage IV colorectal carcinoma clearly benefit from complete resection of hepatic disease. Resection of liver metastases in patients with malignant melanoma and genitourinary cancers, including renal

45

R.K. Yantiss (ed.), *Frozen Section Library: Liver, Extrahepatic Biliary Tree and Gallbladder*, Frozen Section Library, DOI 10.1007/978-1-4614-0043-1_3,
© Springer Science+Business Media, LLC 2011

cell carcinoma, has also met with some success, although data supporting aggressive approaches to these malignancies are not as well established as those for colorectal carcinoma [4]. Metastatic low-to-intermediate grade endocrine neoplasms in the liver may be surgically removed with an intent for cure or to alleviate symptoms related to hormone elaboration, and rare patients are treated with liver transplantation [5–7]. Thus, pathologists may be called upon to provide guidance for the immediate management of surgical patients with hepatic lesions and extrahepatic malignancies. They may be asked to confirm the diagnosis of metastasis in a patient with known extrahepatic cancer and liver tumors, assess the margins of resected metastatic disease, classify unsuspected hepatic lesions encountered during the surgical procedure, and distinguish between a primary and secondary hepatic malignancies (Table 3.1). A comprehensive discussion of all human malignancies that can metastasize to the liver is beyond the scope of this book, but common issues encountered during intraoperative consultations for patients with extrahepatic tumors will be addressed.

METASTATIC COLORECTAL CARCINOMA IN THE LIVER

The most common indication for partial hepatectomy in western countries is resection of metastatic colorectal adenocarcinoma. Up to 25% of patients with colorectal cancer have liver metastases at the time of diagnosis [8]. A subset of these individuals with stage IV disease limited to the liver have prolonged survival following liver resection compared with patients who are not surgically treated [9, 10]. There are two minimal criteria for resection of colorectal cancer metastases in the liver. First, all detectable disease should be resectable, and second, at least 20–30% of the total liver volume should be preserved [11–13]. Fong et al. devised a scoring system to assess resectability of hepatic metastases and predict clinical outcome following surgery for stage IV colorectal carcinoma [14]. This scheme evaluates patients for the presence of five criteria: (1) positive lymph nodes, (2) <12 month disease-free interval between detection of primary tumor and discovery of liver metastases, (3) more than one tumor nodule, (4) preoperative CEA level >200 ng/mL, and (5) largest tumor >5 cm in diameter. When present, each criterion is assigned one point and the values are added to yield a maximum score of five. Colon cancer patients who undergo liver resection and who also do not have any points have a 5-year survival of approximately 60%, whereas patients with five points have a much lower survival of only 14% [14, 15].

The radiographic appearance of metastatic colorectal cancer in the liver is characteristic, so the diagnosis is rarely in question

TABLE 3.1 Features that distinguish primary and secondary malignancies of the liver.

Feature	Hepatocellular carcinoma	Metastatic adenocarcinoma	Metastatic melanoma	Metastatic endocrine tumor
Gross findings				
Tumor number	Solitary > multiple	Multiple > solitary	Multiple	Multiple
Background liver	Cirrhotic	Unremarkable	Unremarkable	Unremarkable
Microscopic findings				
Architecture	Trabeculae Pseudoglands with bile Solid sheets	Irregular glands Single cells Luminal/cellular mucin	Sheets Nests	Nests Trabeculae Glands
Quality of stroma	Absent or minimal stroma Fibrous in some variants	Desmoplastic stroma	Minimal stroma	Hyalinized stroma
Cytology	Uniform cells resembling hepatocytes Pleomorphism in high-grade tumors	Pleomorphic Signet ring cells	Pleomorphic cells Eosinophilic cytoplasm Eccentric nuclei Macronucleoli Melanin pigment	Round cells Eosinophilic cytoplasm Stippled chromatin
Mitoses	Easily detected	Easily detected	Easily detected	Rare/absent

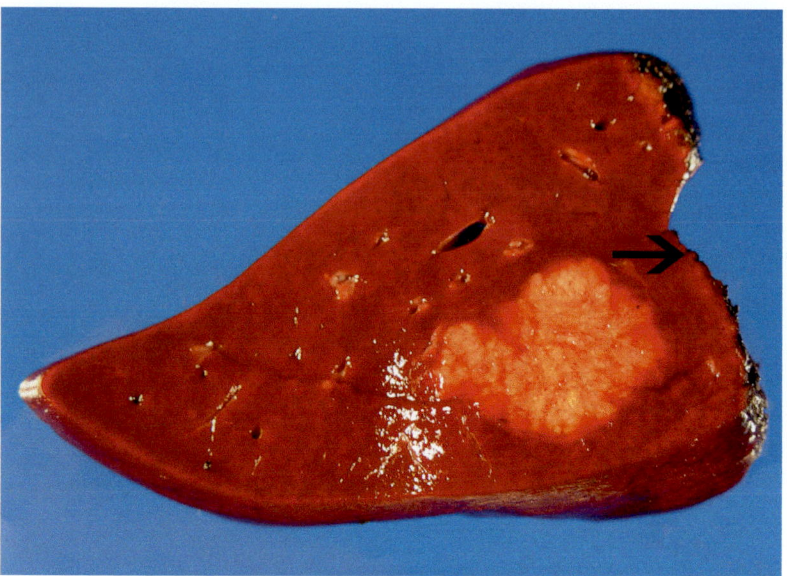

FIG. 3.1 A solitary deposit of metastatic colorectal adenocarcinoma is yellow–white with an ill-defined, loculated border. The tumor is present within 1 cm of the inked resection margin (*arrow*).

at the time of hepatic surgery. Pathologists generally receive a wedge resection, segmentectomy, or more extensive partial hepatectomy specimen with a clearly identifiable cauterized resection margin that is inked prior to sectioning. Gross photographs document the relationship between the tumor and resection margin. The distance from tumor to margin is variable, depending on the nature of the resection specimen, but surgeons try to remove as little nontumoral liver as possible to maximally preserve hepatic function. Sections submitted for frozen section evaluation should be taken perpendicularly to the resection margin and include the tumor, if possible (Fig. 3.1).

Colorectal carcinoma metastases appear as one, or more, ill-defined yellow–white nodules with a scalloped edge. Some tumors have a bilobed, or dumbbell-shaped, appearance that may lead one to erroneously assume a solitary tumor to be multifocal, so review of the radiographic findings prior to evaluating the resection specimen is essential. Metastatic colorectal carcinoma deposits have a depressed, variegated cut surface reflecting extensive necrosis (Fig. 3.2). A variable amount of desmoplastic stroma

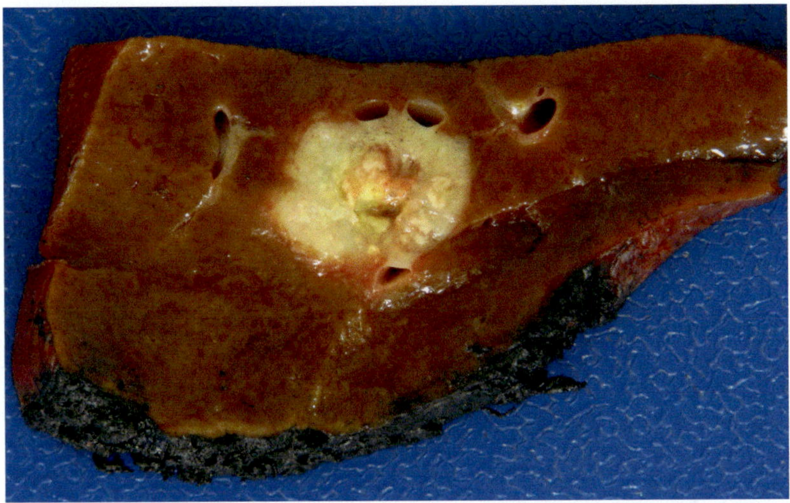

FIG. 3.2 This colorectal adenocarcinoma has a variegated cut surface owing to the presence of central necrosis.

surrounds malignant glands, which characteristically contain necrotic luminal debris (Figs. 3.3 and 3.4). Tumors treated with preoperative systemic chemotherapy or tumor embolization are entirely nonviable or show stromal hyalinization, in which case malignant glands are more numerous peripherally (Fig. 3.5). Treated metastatic deposits should be evaluated for extent of therapeutic response because this finding may be predictive of survival. One should obtain a perpendicular section documenting the relationship between tumor and resection margin and submit a full cross section of the tumor face in multiple cassettes to document the percentage and location of viable carcinoma cells.

ENDOCRINE NEOPLASMS

Liver metastases from endocrine neoplasms may elaborate hormones that are not inactivated *via* the enterohepatic circulation and, thus, produce hormone-related symptoms. Most commonly, metastatic endocrine tumors from the distal small bowel secrete serotonin, resulting in the carcinoid syndrome (i.e., incapacitating episodes of flushing, sweating, and voluminous diarrhea). Patients with metastatic insulin-producing pancreatic endocrine tumors may suffer life-threatening hypoglycemic episodes that are refractory to medical therapy. In these situations, patients could

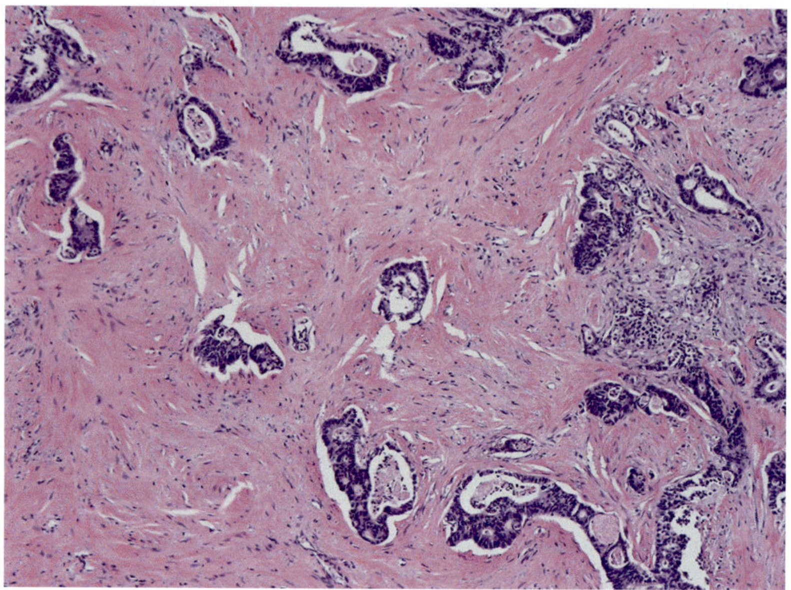

Fig. 3.3 This metastatic colorectal adenocarcinoma contains infiltrative glands with luminal necrosis.

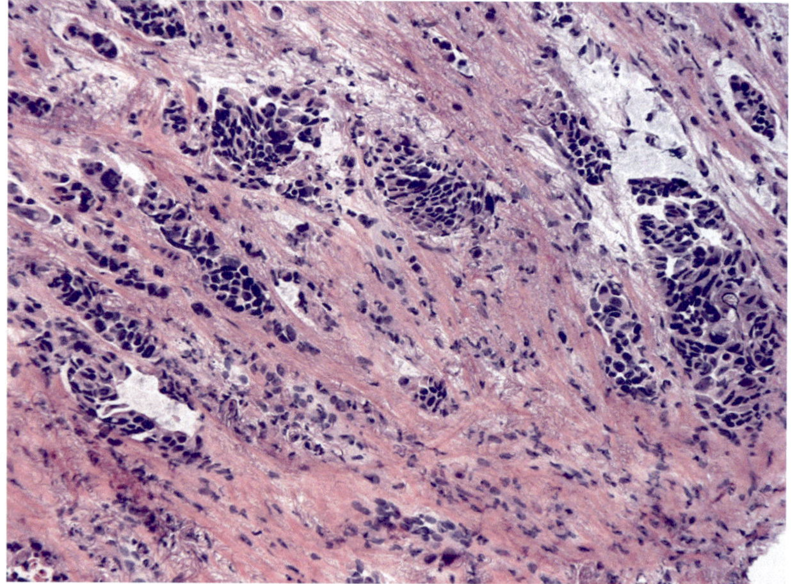

Fig. 3.4 Metastatic colorectal cancer contains glands with marked nuclear variability and hyperchromasia. The glands are associated with desmoplastic stroma.

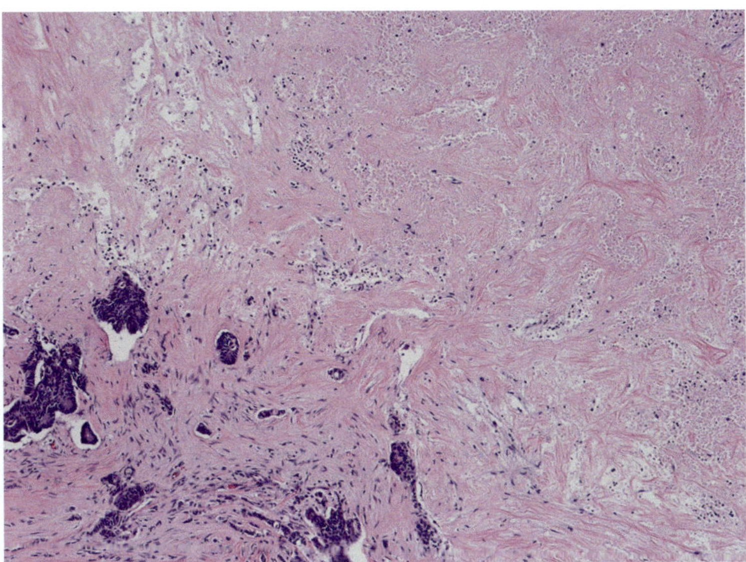

FIG. 3.5 Residual glands of a neoadjuvantly treated rectal carcinoma are located at the tumor periphery. The center of the tumor is necrotic and hyalinized.

be offered surgical resection of hepatic metastases for symptomatic relief. Surgery also prolongs symptom-free survival among patients with limited metastatic disease outside the liver and good performance status [5, 16, 17]. Liver transplantation for patients with metastatic well-differentiated endocrine tumors limited to the liver has met with variable success, although many patients develop relatively rapid disease recurrence that probably results from sustained immunosuppression [18, 19]. Hepatic surgery for endocrine tumors is reserved for patients with well-differentiated (low-to-intermediate grade) tumors because poorly differentiated carcinomas pursue a very aggressive clinical course that is not deterred by surgical intervention. Resection of liver metastases may occur during the removal of the primary tumor or in a subsequent procedure [20]. Thus, discovery of hepatic lesions during resection of the primary neoplasm may prompt an intraoperative consultation when patients do not have previously documented metastases.

Pathologists receive different types of specimens from patients with metastatic endocrine tumors, so understanding the clinical scenario is important. Surgeons may send needle core or wedge biopsy specimens of lesions discovered at the time of surgical exploration, in which case frozen section analysis is performed to make a diagnosis and document the extent of the disease. Solitary tumors,

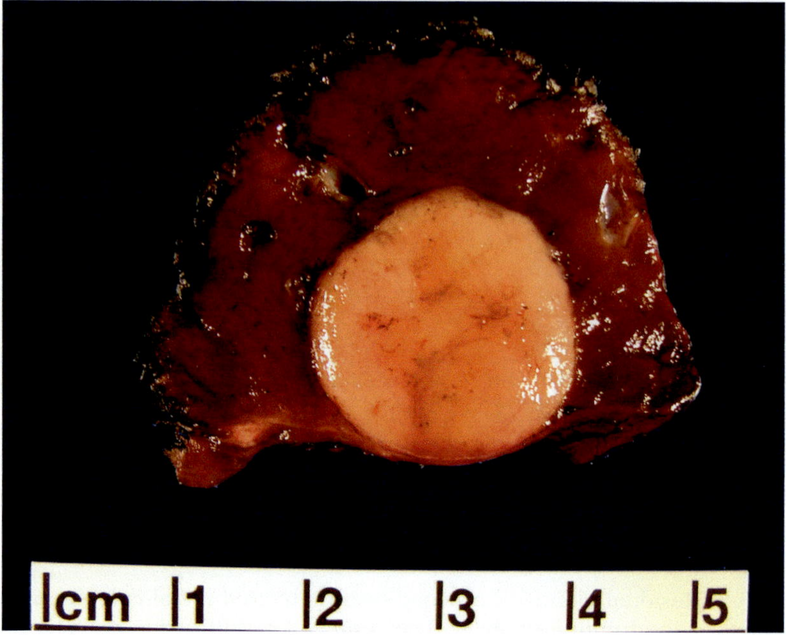

Fɪɢ. 3.6 This metastatic endocrine neoplasm from the small intestine is a well-circumscribed, yellow–white mass that bulges from the cut surface and is present 1 cm from the inked resection margin.

or limited tumor burden, may be resected *in toto*, in which case pathologists are expected to comment on the adequacy of excision and status of the resection margin. Resection specimens are inked along the margin, sectioned perpendicularly to the margin, and photographed (Fig. 3.6). Close margins are evaluated with frozen section analysis. Rare patients undergo hepatic resection for purposes of obtaining fresh tissue for experimental studies, such as vaccine trials or molecular analysis [21]. In this situation, pathologists should clearly communicate with the surgeon regarding the needs of the patient to ensure the appropriate triage of specimens. Only a minimal amount of material is required by pathology for documentation of disease in these cases.

Well-differentiated endocrine neoplasms are circumscribed tumors that bulge from the cut surface of the liver, although large or preoperatively treated tumors may show degenerative changes and necrosis. Metastases from the tubular gut, especially the distal small intestine, colon, and appendix, are yellow or white, whereas those of the duodenum and pancreas vary from yellow to mahogany brown (Fig. 3.7). Well-differentiated tumors are composed of nests and trabeculae containing round cells with

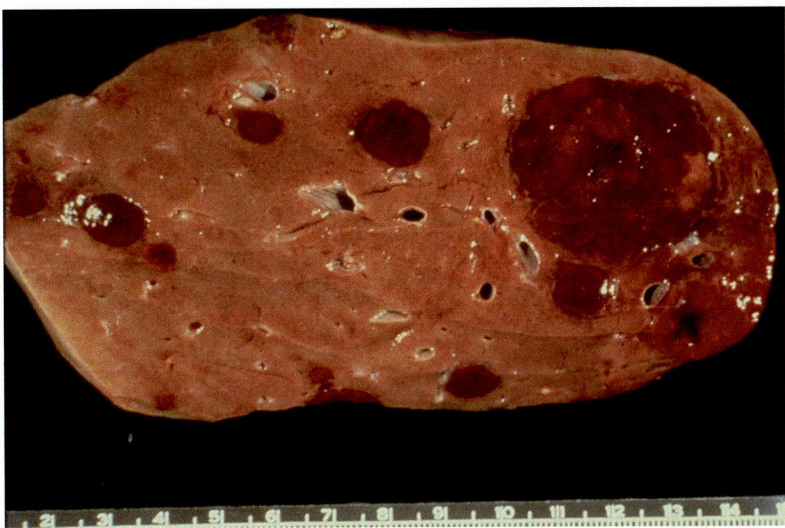

FIG. 3.7 Multiple metastatic tumors from a gastrin-producing duodenal endocrine tumor are circumscribed, red–brown nodules on a background of near-normal liver.

moderate amounts of cytoplasm and round, uniform nuclei (Figs. 3.8 and 3.9). Some tumor cells are pleomorphic with abundant eosinophilic cytoplasm, large, degenerative-appearing nuclei, and nuclear pseudoinclusions. These lesions may simulate adenocarcinoma, particularly when evaluation is limited to needle core biopsy and the tumor contains entrapped bile ducts (Fig. 3.10). Well-differentiated endocrine neoplasms contain round or plasmacytoid cells with abundant eosinophilic cytoplasm (Fig. 3.11). Low-grade neoplasms do not show appreciable mitotic activity or individual cell necrosis, both of which are present to a limited extent in intermediate-grade tumors. Metastatic well-differentiated endocrine tumors typically contain hyalinized stroma that may be a helpful diagnostic clue (Fig. 3.12). This stroma is distinct from the desmoplasia of metastatic carcinoma and the fibrosis of hepatocellular carcinomas, both of which may be considered in the differential diagnosis of metastatic endocrine tumors, particularly when the latter show cellular pleomorphism (Fig. 3.13).

METASTATIC ADENOCARCINOMA

Most hepatic metastases are radiographically evident, so patients are clinically staged prior to resection of the primary tumor. However, some individuals have small liver nodules that escape

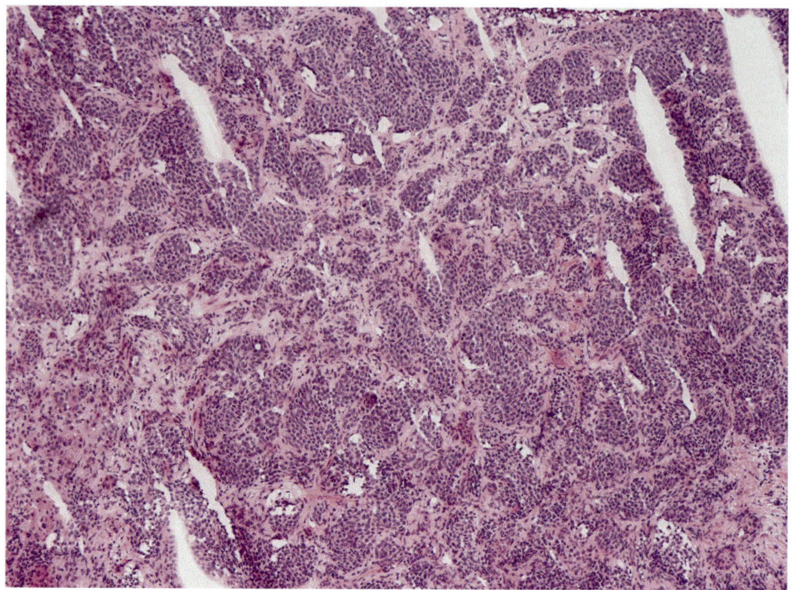

FIG. 3.8 Metastatic well-differentiated endocrine tumors are very cellular and contain tumor cell nests with intervening paucicellular stroma.

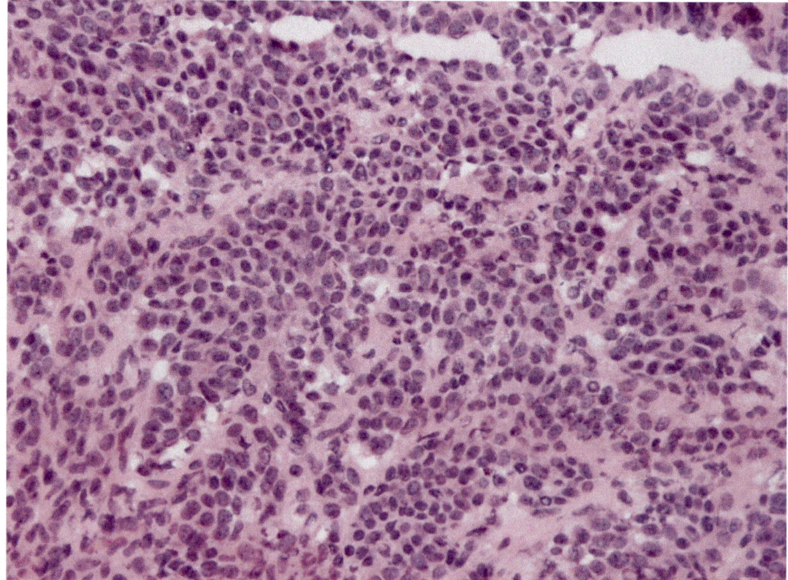

FIG. 3.9 Well-differentiated endocrine tumors contain round nuclei with stippled chromatin and a moderate amount of eosinophilic cytoplasm.

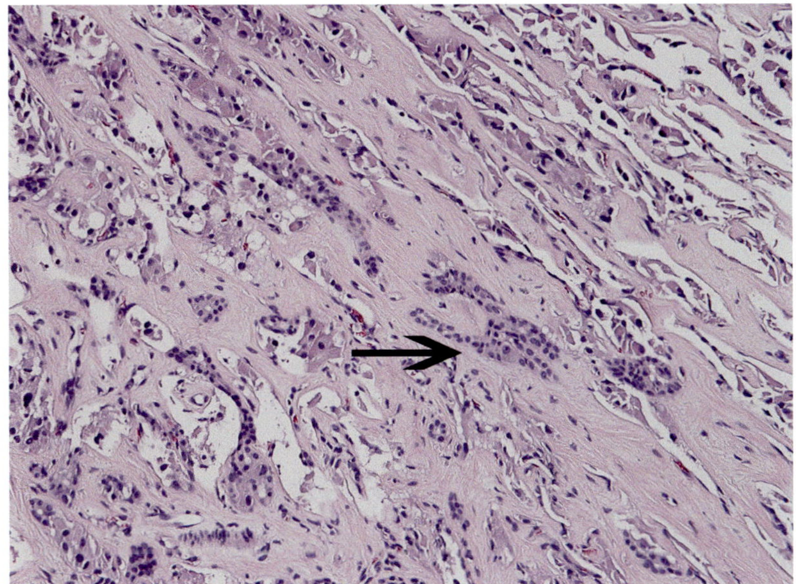

FIG. 3.10 Pleomorphic well-differentiated pancreatic endocrine tumor simulates adenocarcinoma in the liver. The tumor cells are large with ample cytoplasm and atypical nuclei. Entrapped benign bile ducts could be misinterpreted as a glandular component (*arrow*).

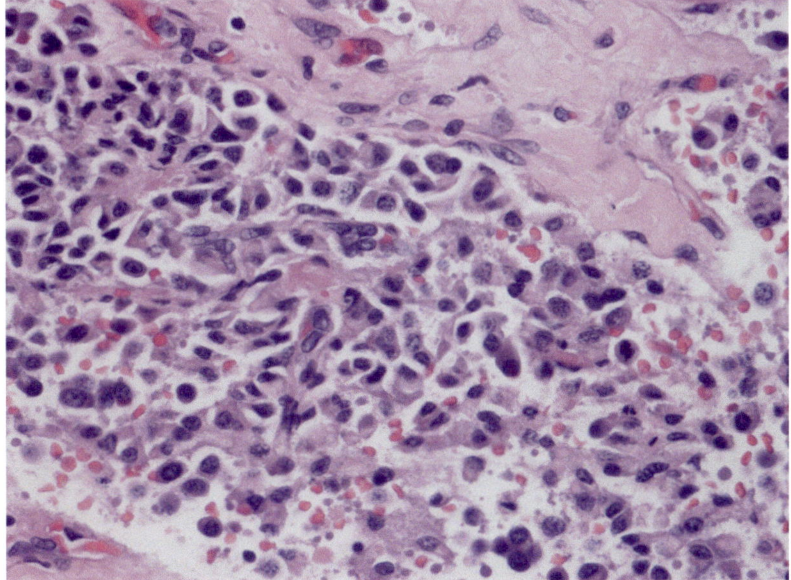

FIG. 3.11 Some metastatic well-differentiated endocrine tumors contain cells with eccentric nuclei and a plasmacytoid appearance.

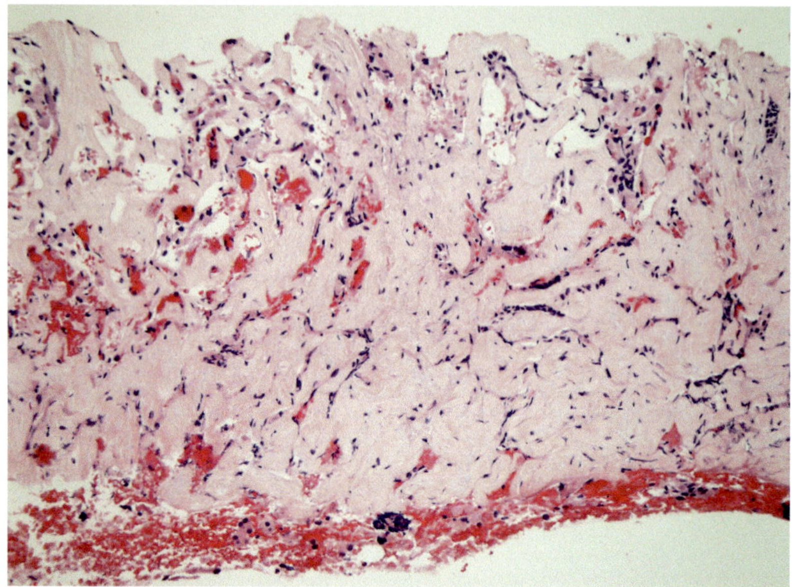

FIG. 3.12 Metastatic endocrine neoplasms contain variable amounts of hyalinized stroma that should be a clue to the diagnosis.

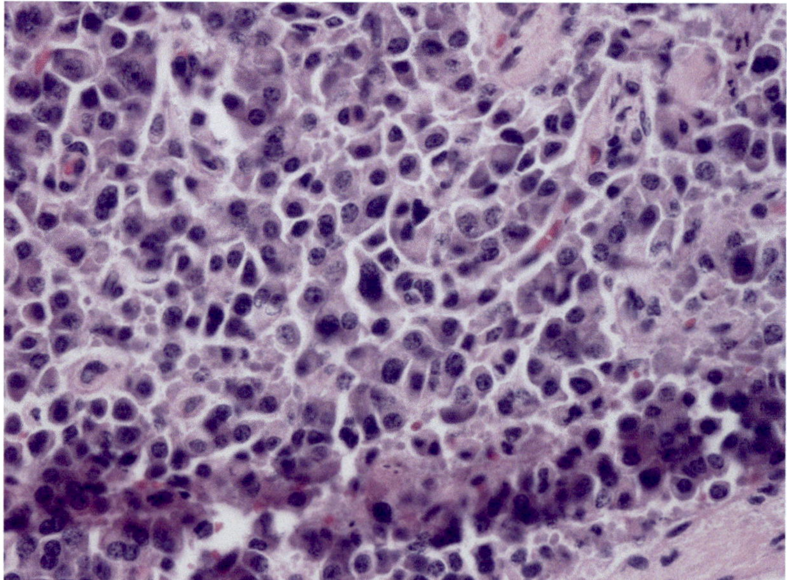

FIG. 3.13 Pleomorphic endocrine tumors contain large atypical cells with irregular nuclei that simulate adenocarcinoma. This tumor is devoid of mitotic activity, despite its worrisome appearance.

radiographic detection. These lesions are discovered during exploratory laparotomy for intra-abdominal malignancies and submitted for frozen section analysis, the results of which will dictate immediate patient management. Adenocarcinomas of the pancreas, extrahepatic bile ducts, gallbladder, esophagus, and stomach are generally considered unresectable if they are associated with liver metastases, thus their distinction from benign biliary lesions of the liver is important. Metastatic adenocarcinomas from the upper gastrointestinal tract and pancreaticobiliary tree are morphologically similar. Most are poorly circumscribed, expansile nodules composed of irregularly spaced, angulated glands associated with desmoplastic stroma (Fig. 3.14). These glands may contain mucin or proteinaceous debris with necrotic cells, but are unassociated with bile (Fig. 3.15). The tumor cell nuclei vary in size, but tend to be enlarged and hyperchromatic with mitotic figures and apoptotic cellular debris (Fig. 3.16). The differential diagnosis of metastatic adenocarcinoma includes bile duct hamartoma (von Meyenberg complex) and bile duct adenoma (biliary adenoma) [22]. Both benign lesions form small, subcapsular nodules that are detected at the time of laparotomy and, thus, their discovery almost always prompts intraoperative consultation. Bile duct hamartomas are rarely confused with carcinoma owing

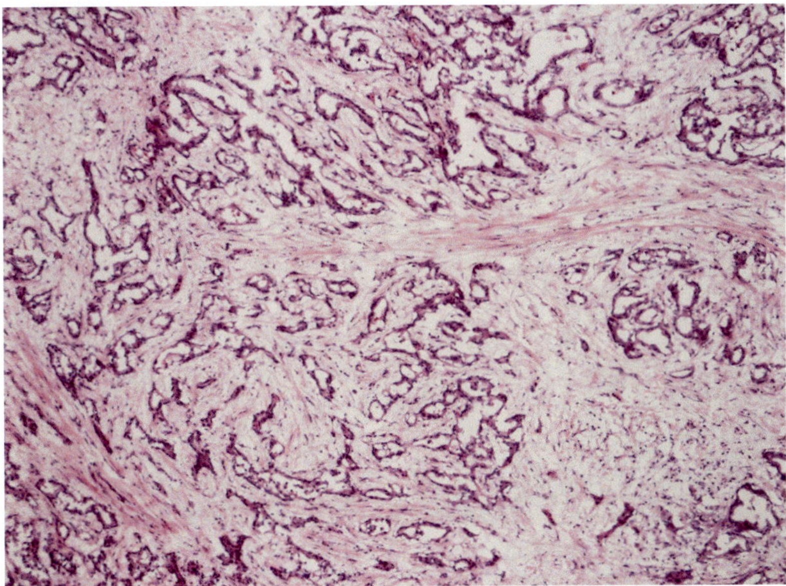

FIG. 3.14 This metastatic pancreatic ductal adenocarcinoma contains irregular aggregates of infiltrative glands. The stroma is desmoplastic.

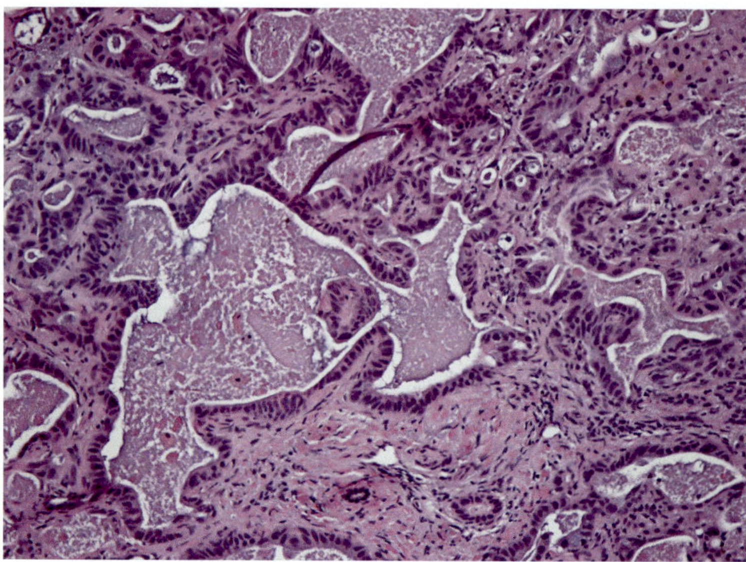

FIG. 3.15 The malignant glands of metastatic pancreatic carcinoma are irregularly-spaced and interconnected. They show variable dilatation with inspissated mucinous material and necrotic cells in gland lumina.

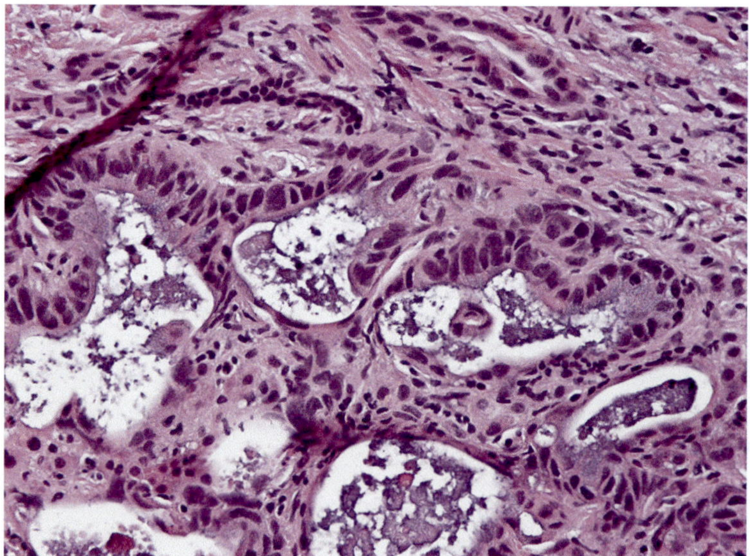

FIG. 3.16 The tumor cells of metastatic pancreatic carcinoma show a high nuclear-to-cytoplasmic ratio, nuclear pleomorphism, and hyperchromasia. The lumina contain necrotic cells and mucin. Note the variability in nuclear size within a single gland.

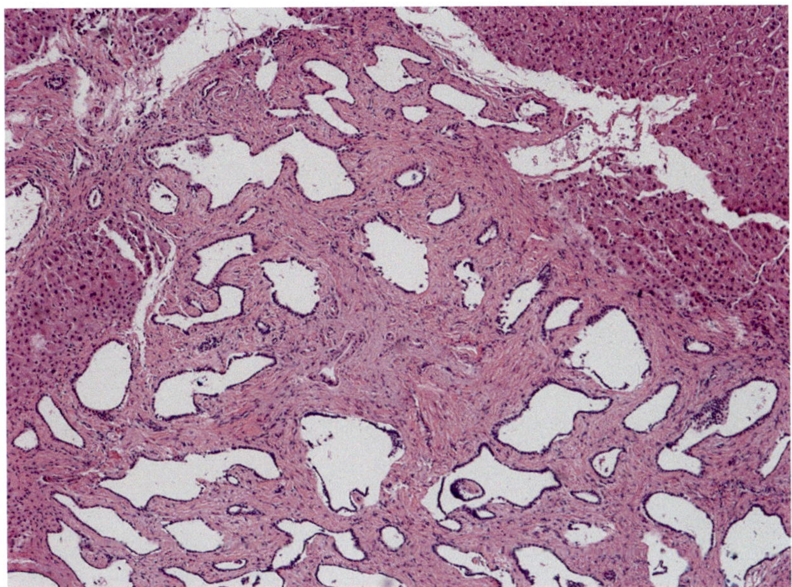

Fɪɢ. 3.17   Bile duct hamartomas are well-circumscribed nodules consisting of cystically dilated glands in dense collagenous stroma. The glands are lined by flattened epithelium.

to their well-circumscribed appearance, hyalinized stroma, and complete lack of cytologic atypia, whereas bile duct adenomas pose several challenges at the time of frozen section (Figs. 3.17 and 3.18). Bile duct hamartomas and bile duct adenomas are discussed in Chapter 2.

METASTATIC NEOPLASMS THAT SIMULATE HEPATOCELLULAR CARCINOMA

A variety of epithelial and nonepithelial malignancies metastasize to the liver where they simulate the appearance of hepatocellular carcinoma. Distinguishing between primary and secondary hepatic tumors is clinically important, since the former may be amenable to surgical resection whereas the latter often are not. The classification of hepatic neoplasms as primary or secondary is usually performed on biopsy material obtained prior to a surgical procedure, although intraoperative consultations may be requested if an extrahepatic malignancy is not suspected prior to exploration. In this situation, evaluating the nonneoplastic liver may be helpful. Most primary hepatic carcinomas occur in association with chronic liver and/or biliary injury, whereas patients

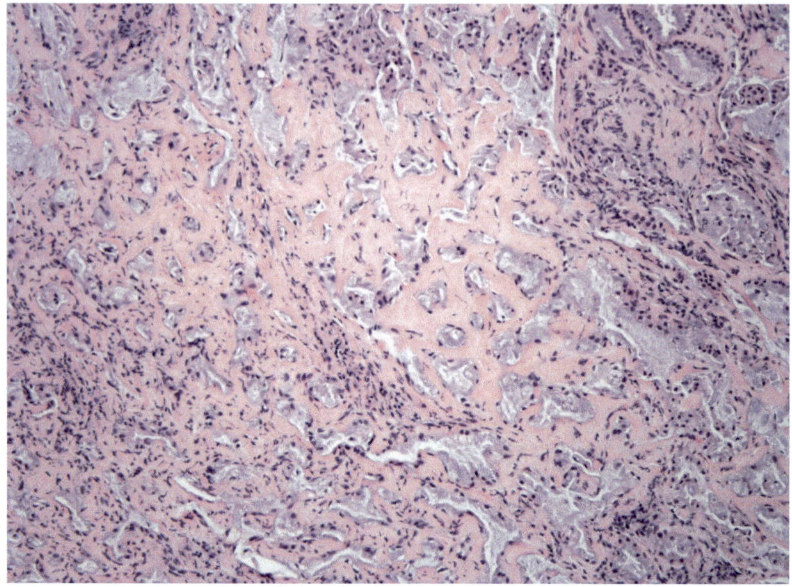

FIG. 3.18 Bile duct adenomas are rounded lesions composed of numerous tubules in cellular stroma. Some tubules contain mucin.

with established cirrhosis and extrahepatic malignancies generally do not develop metastases to the liver. One should always consider the possibility of a metastatic tumor when evaluating a hepatic malignancy that is unassociated with underlying liver disease.

Malignant melanoma frequently metastasizes to the liver, but the diagnosis is often unsuspected because at least one-third develop in patients who do not have a history of malignant melanoma [23–25]. Metastatic deposits are multifocal and extensively replace the hepatic parenchyma (Fig. 3.19). The tumor cells are arranged in organoid nests and "pseudoglandular" or acinar structures that simulate hepatocellular carcinoma (Fig. 3.20). They contain abundant granular eosinophilic cytoplasm and large, eccentric nuclei with macronucleoli (Fig. 3.21). Other neoplasms that mimic hepatocellular carcinoma include adrenal cortical carcinoma, renal chromophobe carcinoma, and pleomorphic endocrine tumors of pancreatic origin (Figs. 3.22 and 3.23). All of these types of tumor may contain polygonal cells with abundant eosinophilic cytoplasm, large nuclei, and prominent nucleoli. Accurate classification may not be possible if evaluation is limited to histologic review, so immunohistochemical stains are generally required (Table 3.2).

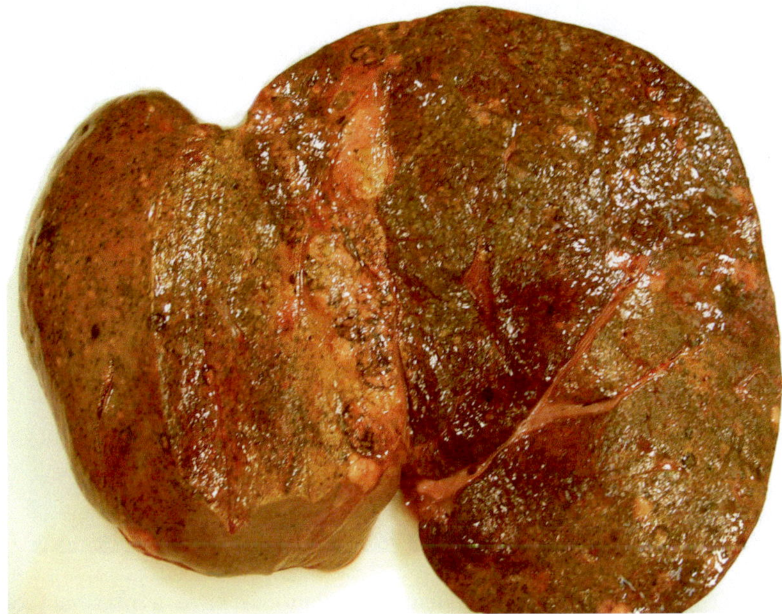

FIG. 3.19 Metastatic malignant melanoma forms multiple variably pigmented nodules that extensively replace the hepatic parenchyma.

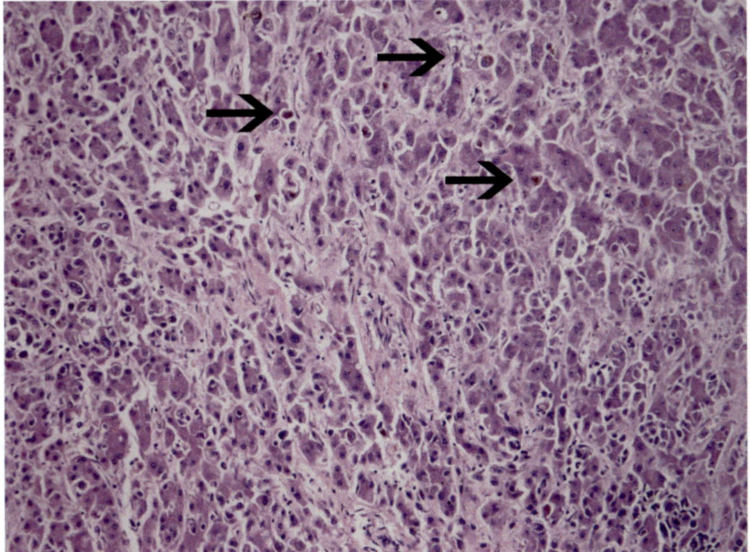

FIG. 3.20 This metastatic melanoma contains nests of dyshesive, highly atypical cells replacing with abundant eosinophilic cytoplasm. Occasional cells contain melanin (*arrow*).

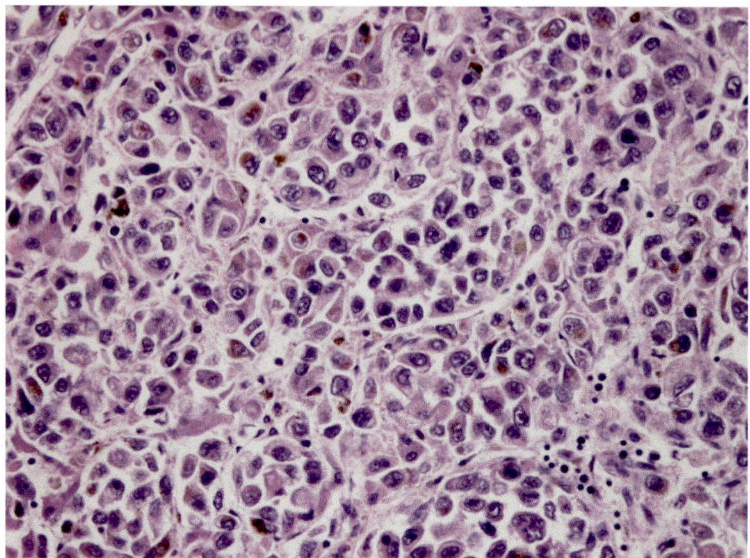

FIG. 3.21 The cells of this metastatic melanoma have a plasmacytoid appearance with pleomorphic, eccentric nuclei and eosinophilic cytoplasm. Cytoplasmic melanin is also present.

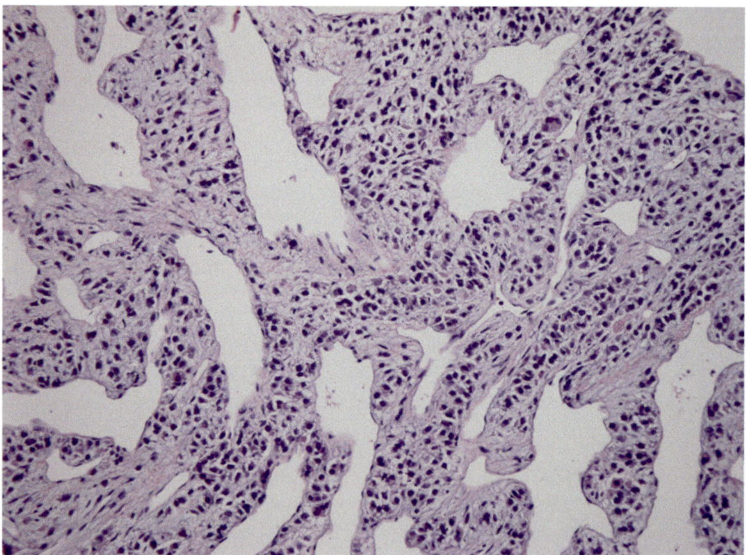

FIG. 3.22 Metastatic adrenal cortical carcinoma contains clear cells with round nuclei separated by dilated vascular spaces. This appearance is reminiscent of clear cell hepatocellular carcinoma with trabecular architecture.

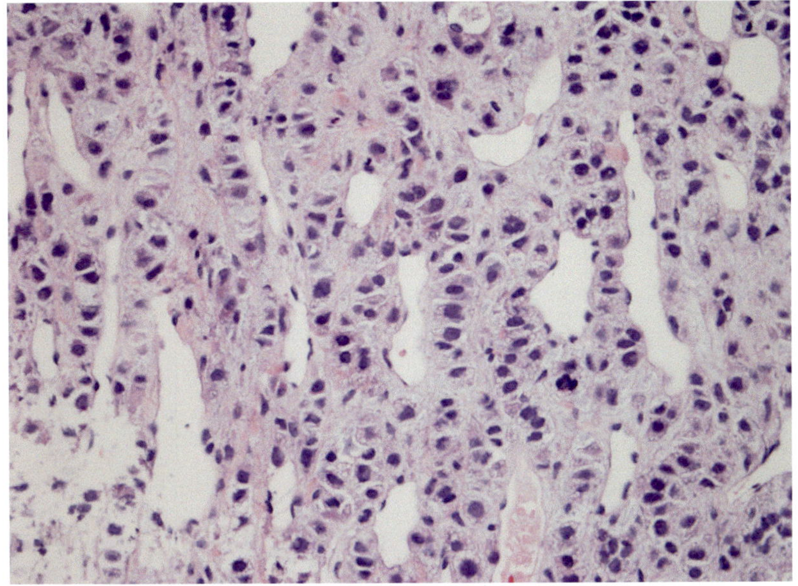

FIG. 3.23 Metastatic adrenal cortical carcinoma contains cells with vacuolated cytoplasm and central nuclei with minimal pleomorphism.

TABLE 3.2 Immunohistochemical features of hepatic tumors that contain cells with eosinophilic cytoplasm.

Immunostain	Hepatocellular carcinoma	Renal cell carcinoma	Adrenal cortical carcinoma	Malignant melanoma	Pancreatic endocrine tumor
Vimentin	Negative	Positive	Negative	Positive	Negative
Cytokeratin 7	Positive	Negative	Negative	Negative	50% positive
Cytokeratin 20	Negative	Negative	Negative	Negative	33% positive
S-100 protein	Negative	Negative	Negative	Positive	Negative
HMB-45	Negative	Negative	Negative	Positive	Negative
A-103	Negative	Negative	Positive	Positive	Negative
CD10	Positive, canalicular pattern	Positive	Negative	Negative	Negative
Inhibin	Negative	Negative	Positive	Negative	Negative
Chromogranin	Negative	Negative	Negative	Negative	Positive

Based on data from: Renshaw and Granter [26]; Murakata et al. [27]; Parwani et al. [28]

References

1. Pickren JW, Tsukada Y, Lane WW. Liver metastases: analysis of autopsy data. In: Weiss L, Gilbert HA, editors. Liver metastases. Boston: Hall Medical Publishers; 1982. p. 2–18.
2. Bhattacharya R, Rao S, Kowdley KV. Liver involvement in patients with solid tumors of nonhepatic origin. Clin Liver Dis. 2002;6(4): 1033–43.
3. Ercolani G, Grazi GL, Ravaiolo M, et al. The role of liver resections for noncolorectal, nonneuroendocrine metastases: experience with 142 observed cases. Ann Surg Oncol. 2005;12:459–66.
4. Staehler MD, Kruse J, Haseke N, et al. Liver resection for metastatic disease prolongs survival in renal cell carcinoma: 12-year results from a retrospective comparative analysis. World J Urol. 2010;28:543–7.
5. Boleslawski E, Dharancy S, Truant S, Pruvot FR. Surgical management of liver metastases from gastrointestinal endocrine tumors. Gastroentérol Clin Biol. 2010;34(4–5):274–82.
6. Reddy SK, Clary BM. Neuroendocrine liver metastases. Surg Clin North Am. 2010;90(4):853–61.
7. Hwang S, Lee YJ, Lee SG, et al. Surgical treatment of primary neuroendocrine tumors of the liver. J Gastrointest Surg. 2008;12(4): 725–30.
8. Yang A, Brouquet A, Vauthey J. Extending limits of resection for metastasis of colorectal cancer: risk benefit ratio. J Surg Oncol. 2010;102(8):996–1001.
9. Scheele J, Stangle R, Altendorf-Hofmann A. Hepatic metastases from colorectal carcinoma: impact of surgical resection on the natural history. Br J Surg. 1990;77(11):1241–6.
10. Lewis AM, Martin RC. The treatment of hepatic metastases in colorectal carcinoma. Am Surg. 2006;72:466–73.
11. Feroci F, Fong Y. Use of clinical score to stage and predict outcome of hepatic resection of metastatic colorectal cancer. J Surg Oncol. 2010;102(8):914–21.
12. Abdalla EK, Adam R, Bilchik AJ, Jaeck D, Vauthey JN, Mahvi D. Improving resectability of hepatic colorectal metastases: expert consensus statement. Ann Surg Oncol. 2006;13:1271–80.
13. Pawlik TM, Choti MA. Surgical therapy for colorectal metastases to the liver. J Gastrointest Surg. 2007;11:1057–77.
14. Fong Y, Fortner J, Sun RL, et al. Clinical score for predicting recurrence after hepatic resection for metastatic colorectal cancer, analysis of 1001 consecutive cases. Ann Surg. 1999;230:309–21.
15. House MG, Ito H, Gonen M, et al. Survival after hepatic resection for colorectal cancer: trends in outcomes for 1,600 patients during two decades at a single institution. J Am Coll Surg. 2010;210(5):744–52.
16. Sarmiento JM, Que FG. Hepatic surgery for metastases from neuroendocrine tumors. Surg Oncol Clin N Am. 2003;12(1):231–42.
17. Glazer ES, Tseng JF, Al-Refaie W, et al. Long-term survival after surgical management of neuroendocrine hepatic metastases. HPB. 2010;12(6):427–33.

18. Marin C, Robles R, Fernandez JA, et al. Role of liver transplantation in the management of unresectable neuroendocrine liver metastases. Transplant Proc. 2007;39(7):2302–3.
19. van Vilsteren FG, Baskin-Bey ES, Nagorney DM, et al. Liver transplantation for gastroenteropancreatic neuroendocrine cancers: defining selection criteria to improve survival. Liver Transpl. 2006; 12(3):448–56.
20. Frilling A, Li J, Malamutmann E, Schmid KW, Bockisch A, Broelsch CE. Treatment of liver metastases from neuroendocrine tumours in relation to the extent of hepatic disease. Br J Surg. 2009;96:175–84.
21. Schulze T, Kemmner W, Weitz J, Wernecke KD, Schirrmacher V, Schlag PM. Efficiency of adjuvant active specific immunization with Newcastle disease virus modified tumor cells in colorectal cancer patients following resection of liver metastases: results of a prospective randomized trial. Cancer Immunol Immunother. 2009;58(1):61–9.
22. Fritz S, Hacker T, Blaker H, et al. Multiple von Meyenberg complexes mimicking diffuse liver metastases from esophageal squamous cell carcinoma. World J Gastroenterol. 2006;12(26):4250–2.
23. Tassier DJ, McConnell EJ, Young-Fadok T, Wolff BG. Melanoma metastatic to the colon: case series and review of the literature with outcome analysis. Dis Colon Rectum. 2003;46(4):441–7.
24. Fusasaki T, Narita R, Hiura M, et al. Acute hepatic failure secondary to extensive hepatic replacement by metastatic amelanotic melanoma: an autopsy report. Clin J Gastroenterol. 2010;6:327–31.
25. Liang KV, Sanderson SO, Nowakowski GS, Arora AS. Metastatic malignant melanoma of the gastrointestinal tract. Mayo Clin Proc. 2006;81(4):511–6.
26. Renshaw A, Granter S. A comparison of A103 and inhibin reactivity in adrenal cortical tumors: distinction from hepatocellular carcinoma and renal tumors. Mod Pathol. 1998;11:1160–4.
27. Murakata L, Ishak K, Nzeako U. Clear cell carcinoma of the liver: a comparative immunohistochemical study with renal clear cell carcinoma. Mod Pathol. 2000;13:874–81.
28. Parwani AV, Chan TY, Mathew S, Ali SZ. Metastatic malignant melanoma in liver aspirate: cytomorphologic distinction from hepatocellular carcinoma. Diagn Cytopathol. 2004;30(4):247–50.

Chapter 4
Mesenchymal and Pediatric Tumors of the Liver

INTRODUCTION

Mesenchymal neoplasms of the liver are uncommon and account for approximately 3% of the primary hepatic neoplasms [1]. Those that develop in adults consist entirely of mesenchymal elements and show a spectrum of morphologic features, including both spindle cell and epithelioid cell morphology. Tumors composed predominantly of epithelioid cells are commonly mistaken for either hepatocellular carcinoma or metastatic adenocarcinoma, especially when evaluated by needle biopsy analysis in either the preoperative or intraoperative setting. Unlike carcinomas, however, most hepatic mesenchymal tumors are either benign or low-grade malignant and, thus, they tend to be amenable to surgery. Primary high-grade sarcomas of the liver are exceedingly uncommon and overtly malignant spindle cell tumors in the liver usually represent metastases. Most pediatric mesenchymal tumors contain mixed mesenchymal and epithelial cell elements and may be either benign or malignant. The majority are amenable to surgical resection despite the fact that they may be quite large.

Intraoperative evaluation of mesenchymal liver tumors is generally performed for one of two reasons. First, surgeons may request frozen section analysis to assess the adequacy of tumor resection. In this situation, the submitted specimen consists of a liver wedge, segmentectomy, or larger resection specimen that contains the tumor. The parenchymal margin is inked and the liver is sectioned perpendicularly to the margin. Gross photographs are obtained to document the relationship between tumor and margin.

67

R.K. Yantiss (ed.), *Frozen Section Library: Liver, Extrahepatic Biliary Tree and Gallbladder*, Frozen Section Library, DOI 10.1007/978-1-4614-0043-1_4,
© Springer Science+Business Media, LLC 2011

Second, pathologists may be called upon to classify tumors when a preoperative diagnosis is not established, or in doubt. Specimens obtained for this purpose are usually needle core biopsies or wedge resections that represent a small sample of a much larger mass. Pathologists should be aware of the clinical scenario before submitting all of a biopsy sample for frozen section analysis, so that some of the material is available for permanent sections and ancillary studies, if necessary.

ANGIOMYLIPOMA

Hepatic angiomyolipoma is an uncommon neoplasm and member of the perivascular epithelioid cell (PEComa) family of mesenchymal tumors, which also includes pulmonary lymphangioleiomyomatosis and clear cell sugar tumors of lung and pancreas. These tumors share a characteristic immunophenotype, namely, strong positivity for HMB45 and melan-A [2]. Most angiomyolipomas occur in the kidney, followed in frequency by the liver, other viscera, and soft tissues. Although renal angiomyolipomas represent one manifestation of tuberous sclerosis, hepatic tumors do not occur in association with this syndrome. Hepatic angiomyolipomas show a strong female predominance and are benign, despite their occasional multicentricity in the liver and perihepatic lymph nodes [2, 3].

Hepatic angiomyolipomas are well-circumscribed tumors with a heterogeneous cut surface reflecting variable amounts of smooth muscle and fat. Grossly visible fat is less prominent in hepatic tumors compared with those of the kidney, and some liver lesions are quite myxoid (Fig. 4.1). Intersecting fascicles of plump smooth muscle cells admixed with mature adipocytes and thick-walled, hyalinized blood vessels are characteristic of renal tumors, but comprise a minority of the tumor volume in hepatic lesions (Fig. 4.2). Rather, angiomyolipomas of the liver contain sheets of epithelioid cells with abundant granular cytoplasm, round nuclei, and prominent nucleoli (Fig. 4.3). Some tumors display nuclear pleomorphism that simulates the appearance of HCC (Fig. 4.4). Mitotic figures and necrosis are infrequent. Large dilated vessels are readily identified (Fig. 4.5).

The distinction between hepatic angiomyolipoma and HCC may be challenging, especially when the frozen section slide contains a predominantly epithelioid cell population and very little fat (Table 4.1). However, the correct diagnosis is usually attainable, or may be suspected, if attention is paid to any one of the several clues. Some hepatocellular carcinomas contain fat

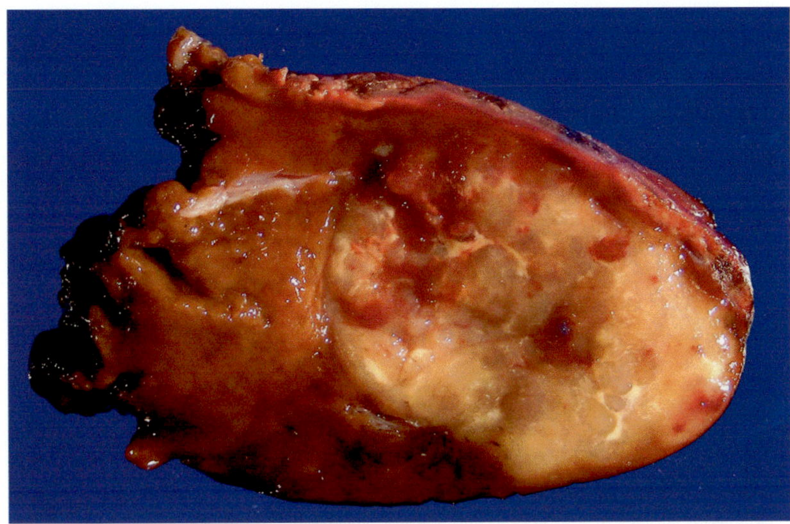

FIG. 4.1 This hepatic angiomyolipoma is well-circumscribed and myxoid with a yellow cut surface. The inked margin is to the *left*.

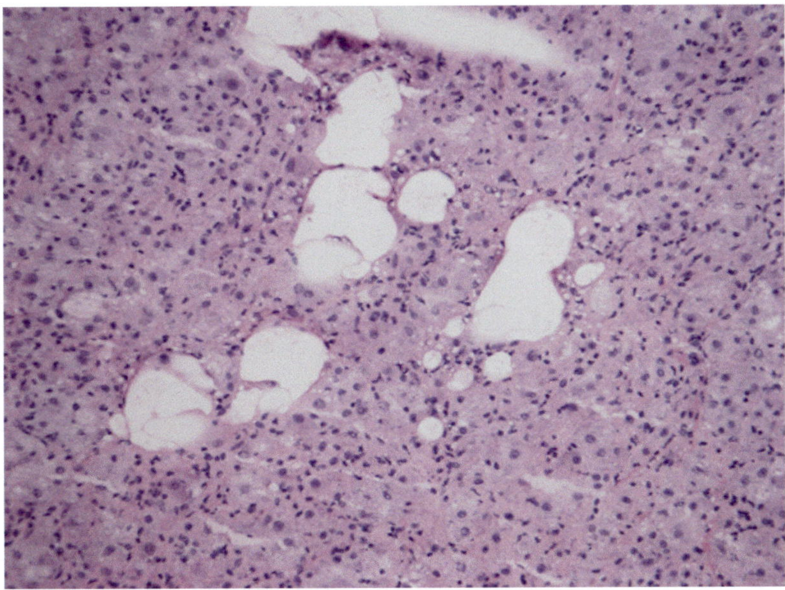

FIG. 4.2 This angiomyolipoma is composed of epithelioid cells with abundant pink cytoplasm admixed with mature adipocytes.

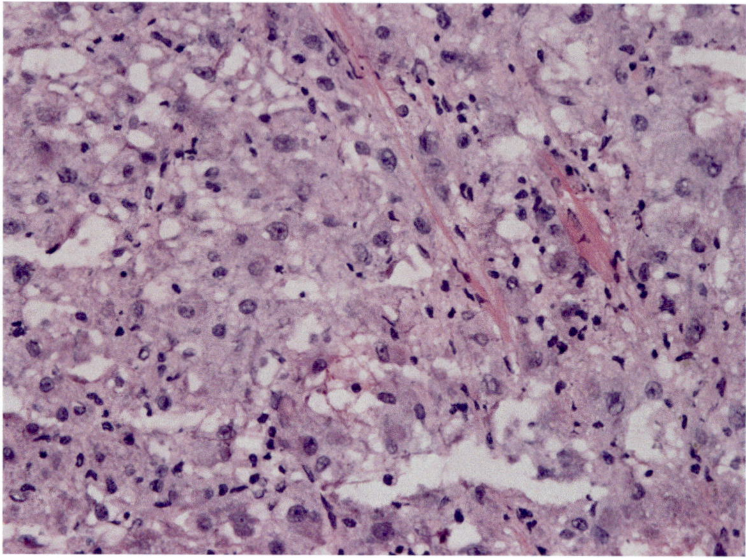

Fɪɢ. 4.3 Epithelioid cells predominate in this hepatic angiomyolipoma. They are round with central nuclei and abundant faintly eosinophilic cytoplasm.

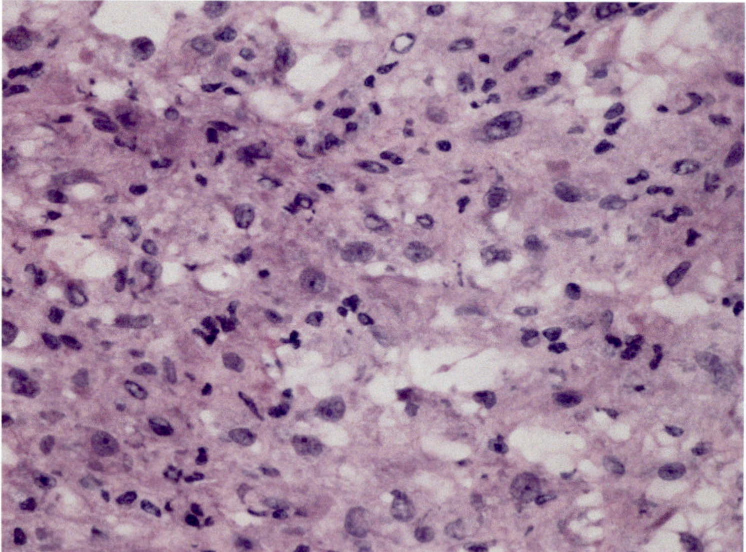

Fɪɢ. 4.4 Angiomyolipomas contain occasional cells with enlarged nuclei and conspicuous nucleoli that simulate the features of hepatocellular carcinoma.

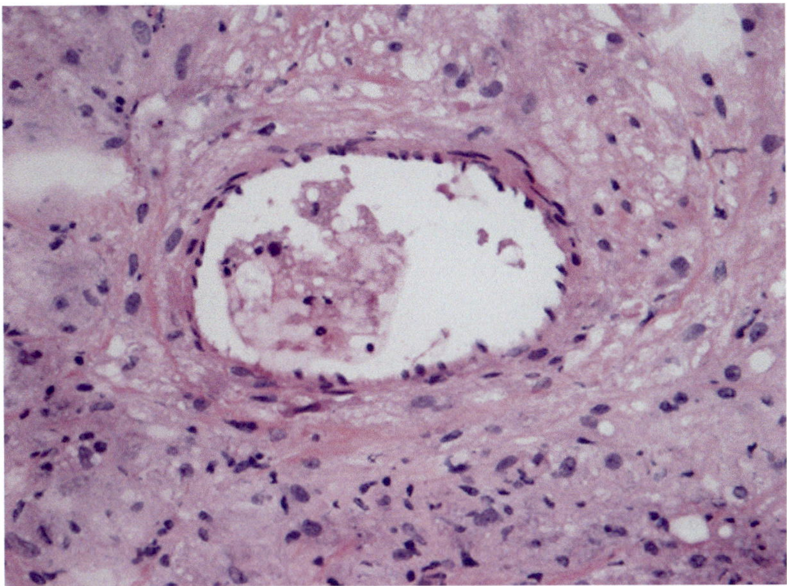

FIG. 4.5 Large vessels surrounded by epithelioid cells are readily identified in an angiomyolipoma.

within tumor cells, but aggregates of mature adipocytes do not occur in HCC unless the tumor has extended beyond the hepatic capsule and invaded soft tissues. Spindle cells are exceedingly rare in HCC and, if present, represent a minor component of a high-grade tumor, which usually shows other features of malignancy, such as tumor necrosis and brisk mitotic activity. Thus, spindle cells in an otherwise bland tumor should lead one away from a diagnosis of HCC. Angiomyolipomas characteristically contain epithelioid cells arranged in sheets and nodules in combination with irregular, dilated thin-walled vascular spaces, but they do not display pseudoglandular or trabecular growth patterns. Nuclear pleomorphism is prominent in some cases, but angiomyolipomas do not display appreciable mitotic activity, cellular necrosis, or any other feature of malignancy. Finally, the clinical features of hepatic angiomyolipomas are distinct from those of most HCCs. Angiomyolipomas tend to occur in young adult women who do not have underlying liver disease, whereas HCCs are more common among older men with cirrhosis.

TABLE 4.1 Distinguishing features of angiomyolipoma and hepatocellular carcinoma.

Feature	Angiomyolipoma	Hepatocellular carcinoma
Clinical features		
Patient age	Mean: 45 years	Mean: 65 years
Patient gender	Male < female	Male > female
Gross features		
Underlying liver disease	Absent	Present
Centricity	Solitary > multiple	Solitary > multiple
Appearance	Heterogeneous with myxoid and yellow areas, cysts, and fat	Brown or green nodule
Microscopic features		
Thick-walled blood vessels	Present Surrounded by condensed tumor cells	Generally absent
Epithelioid cells		
Cytoplasm	Granular, faintly eosinophilic	Dense, hard eosinophilic
Cytoplasmic material	Absent	Fat, bile, hyaline globules
Nuclei	Eccentric with smooth contours	Central and irregular
Mitoses	Absent	Present
Spindle cells	Present	Absent
Tumor fat	Present in adipocytes	Present as vacuoles in tumor cells

VASCULAR TUMORS

Hemangioma

Hemangiomas are among the most common hepatic tumors and certainly the most frequently encountered mesenchymal lesions of the liver [4]. Most occur in young adult females, in whom they may grow under the influence of oral contraceptive pills. The radiographic features of hepatic hemangiomas are quite characteristic, so the diagnosis is usually made without tissue biopsy or resection [5]. The pathologic features of hemangiomas are variable and depend upon the extent of hyalinization present in the tumor stroma. They may be well-circumscribed, soft hemorrhagic nodules composed of irregular thin-walled vascular spaces lined by cytologically bland flattened endothelial cells (Figs. 4.6 and 4.7).

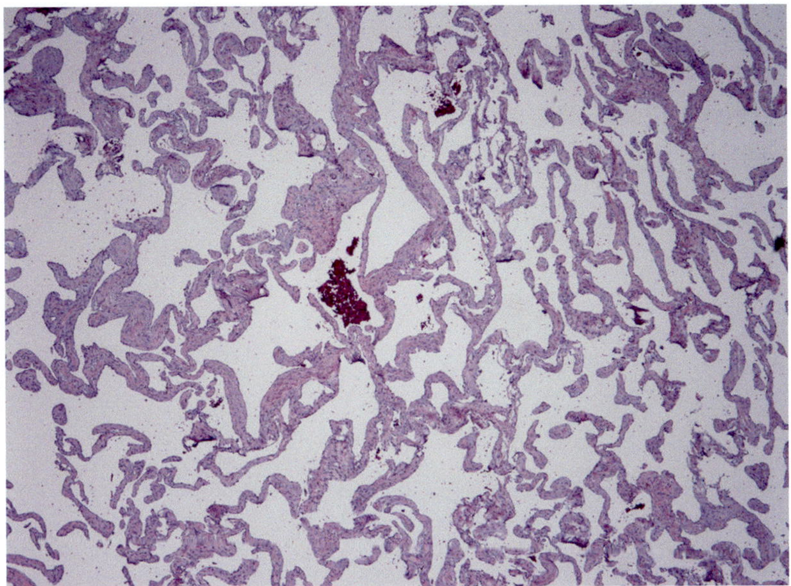

FIG. 4.6   Hemangiomas contain dilated vascular channels with thin septa.

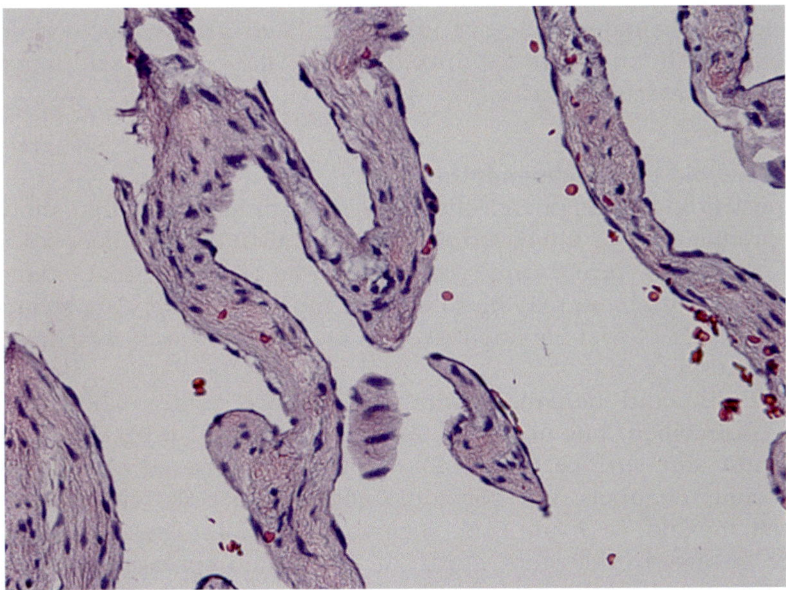

FIG. 4.7   Flat, cytologically bland endothelial cells line the vascular spaces of a hemangioma. The septa are paucicellular.

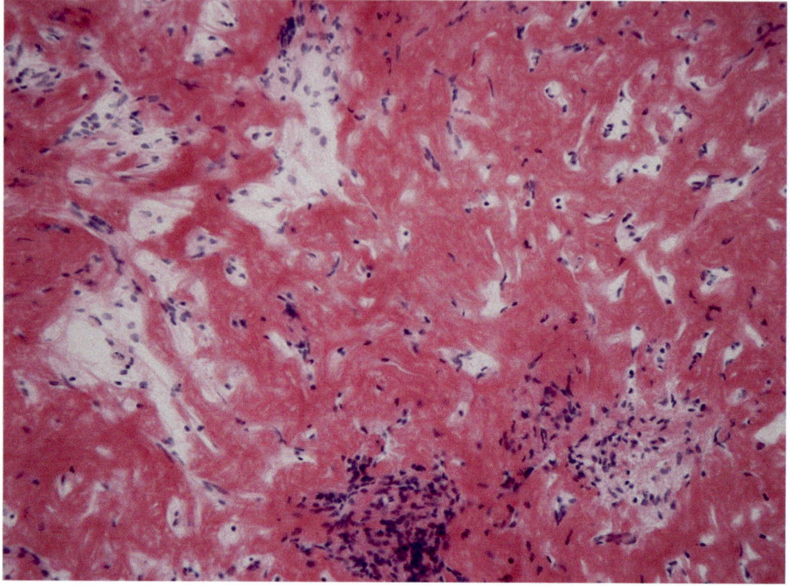

FIG. 4.8 Sclerotic hemangiomas contain ill-defined dense hyalinized collagen that compresses vascular spaces.

Sclerotic hemangiomas are unencapsulated gray–white nodules that contain abundant hyalinized stroma and compressed, inconspicuous vascular spaces (Fig. 4.8).

Epithelioid Hemangioendothelioma

Epithelioid hemangioendothelioma is a rare neoplasm that shows a predilection to affect women in the fourth to fifth decades of life [6]. These tumors are considered to be of intermediate malignant potential and may be solitary or multifocal. They are treated with either partial hepatic resection or, in some cases, liver transplantation [7–9].

Epithelioid hemangioendotheliomas are yellow–white, well circumscribed, but unencapsulated, tumors that bulge from the hepatic cut surface (Fig. 4.9). They are composed of abortive vascular channels and polygonal endothelial cells within abundant myxoid, or hyalinized, stroma (Fig. 4.10). The tumor cells are arranged in clusters, cords, or singly, and contain abundant, faintly eosinophilic cytoplasm (Fig. 4.11). Cytoplasmic vacuoles representing intracellular lumina are usually present, some of which contain red cells, red cell fragments, or eosinophilic globules

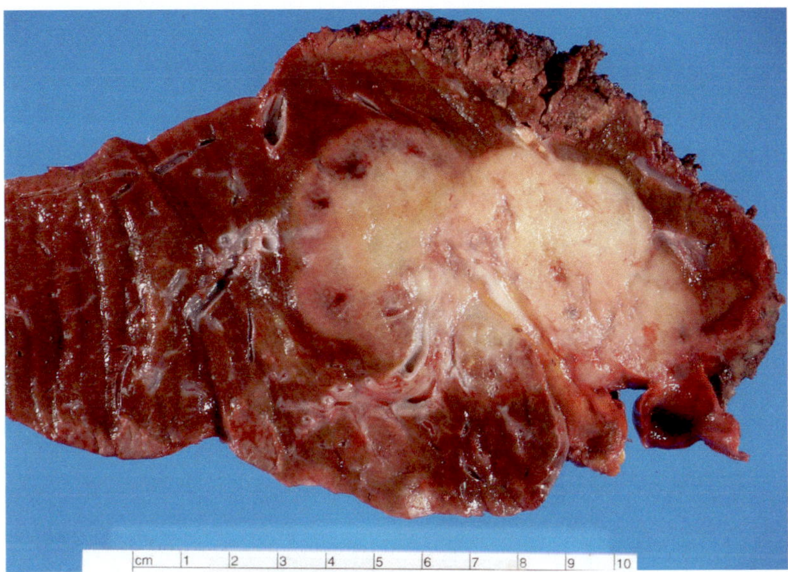

FIG. 4.9 An epithelioid hemangioendothelioma is well-demarcated from the normal background liver. The tumor has a homogeneous pale-yellow cut surface.

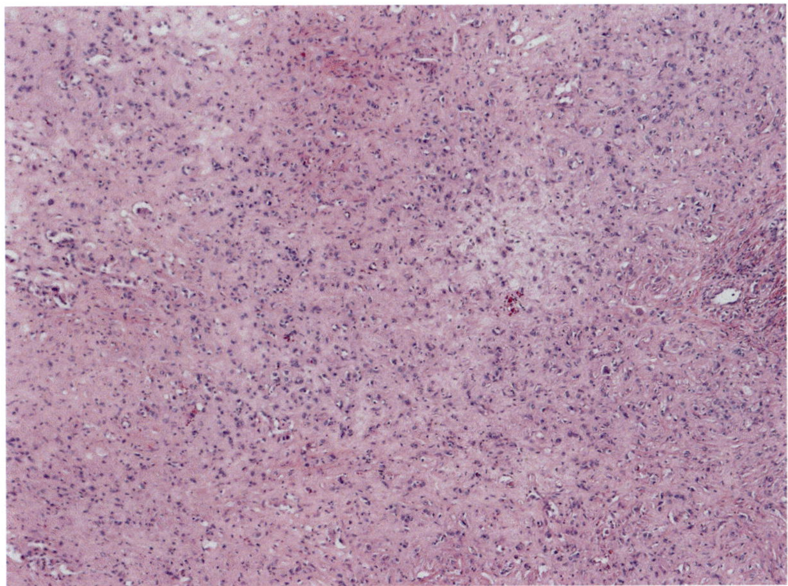

FIG. 4.10 Epithelioid hemangioendotheliomas are variably cellular tumors with hyalinized stroma.

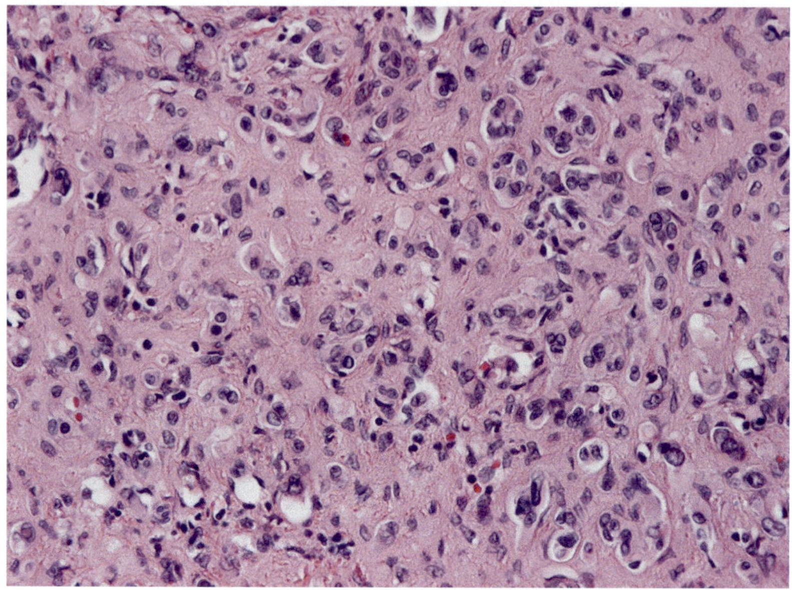

FIG. 4.11 Endothelial cells are arranged in small clusters in this epithelioid hemangioendothelioma. The tumor stroma is hyalinized.

(Fig. 4.12). Cytoplasmic lumina compress the nuclei imparting a signet ring cell appearance to the tumor cells (Fig. 4.13). Occasional mitotic figures are encountered. Notably, tumor foci in adjacent hepatic parenchyma are centered on large vessels with thromboses and projections into the lumen.

Epithelioid hemangioendotheliomas mimic the histologic appearance of metastatic adenocarcinoma. The cytoplasmic lumina closely simulate mucin vacuoles, although carcinomas generally show a greater degree of cytologic atypia (Fig. 4.14). Some tumors contain entrapped benign bile ducts that may be misinterpreted as glandular elements of adenocarcinoma (Fig. 4.15). Features that should lead one to suspect a diagnosis of epithelioid hemangioendothelioma include the presence of paucicellular myxoid or hyalinized stroma, rather than the desmoplastic stroma of metastatic carcinoma. The tumor cells of epithelioid hemangioendothelioma contain sharply demarcated cytoplasmic vacuoles that are distinct from the bubbly cytoplasmic mucin of signet ring cell carcinoma and they generally show less nuclear pleomorphism and mitotic activity than would be expected of adenocarcinoma. Detection of intracytoplasmic lumina containing red blood cells is very helpful in distinguishing between these entities (Table 4.2) [10].

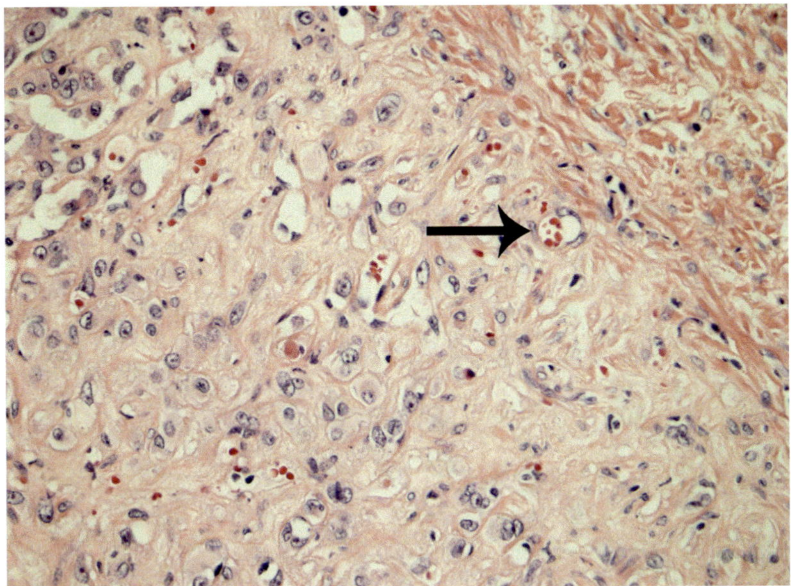

FIG. 4.12 The tumor cells of epithelioid hemangioendothelioma contain intracytoplasmic lumina that represent abortive vascular spaces. Some of the lumina are filled with blood (*arrow*).

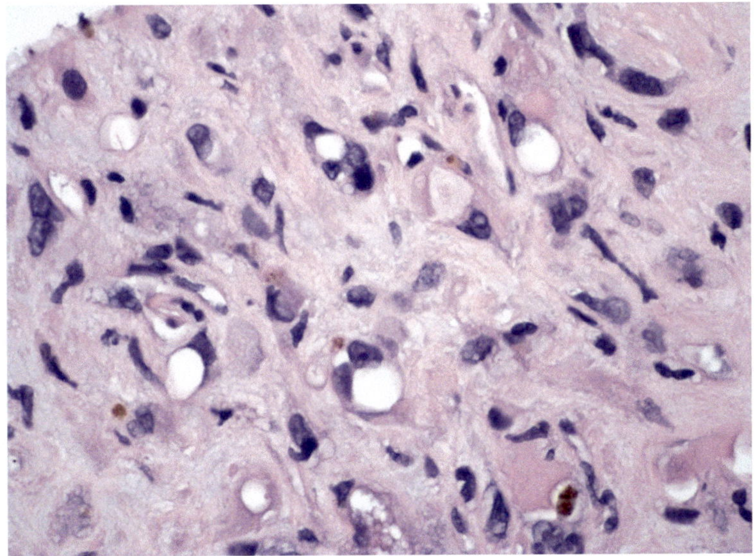

FIG. 4.13 Intracytoplasmic lumina of an epithelioid hemangioendothelioma mimic mucin vacuoles of signet ring cell carcinoma. However, the lumina are optically clear and contain eosinophilic globules that represent red blood cell fragments.

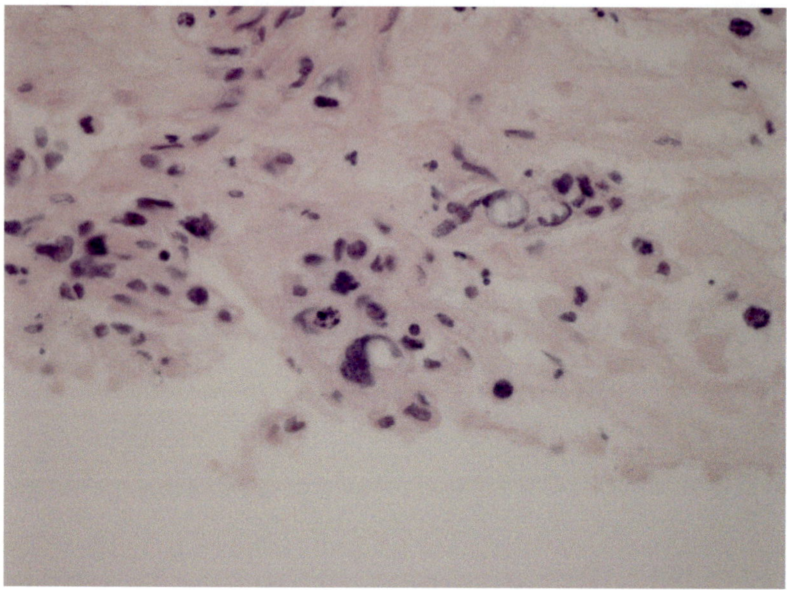

FIG. 4.14 Metastatic pancreatic adenocarcinoma may simulate epithelioid hemangioendothelioma owing to the presence of single cells and signet ring cells within eosinophilic stroma. However, the cytoplasm of these tumor cells is mucinous and the cells are quite atypical.

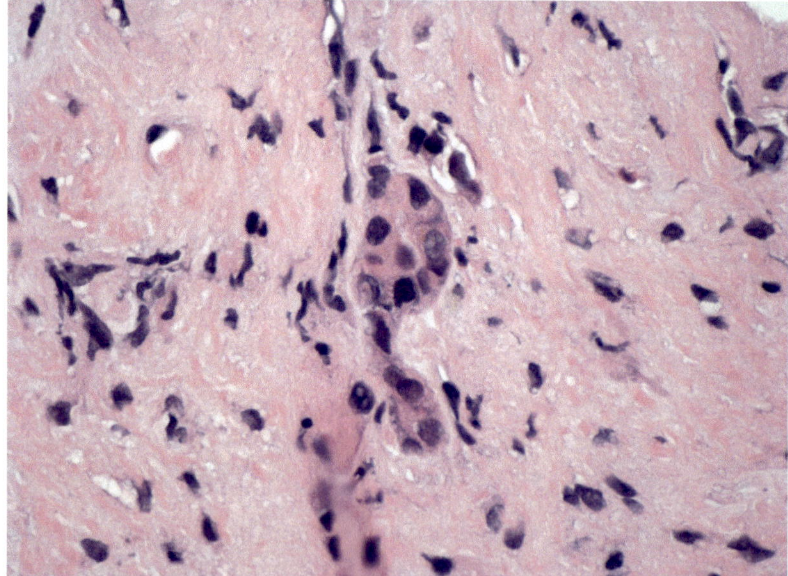

FIG. 4.15 Entrapped bile ducts within an epithelioid hemangioendothelioma simulate the appearance of adenocarcinoma.

TABLE 4.2 Distinguishing features of epithelioid hemangioendothelioma and metastatic adenocarcinoma.

Feature	Epithelioid hemangioendothelioma	Metastatic adenocarcinoma
Clinical features		
Patient age	Mean: 40 years	Mean: 65 years
Gross features		
Underlying liver disease	Absent	Absent
Centricity	Multiple or solitary	Multiple > solitary
Appearance	Well-circumscribed Firm, white	Ill-defined Firm, white
Microscopic features		
Gland formation	Absent	Present
Tumor cell morphology	Epithelioid	Epithelioid
Cytoplasmic vacuoles	Intracytoplasmic lumina with red cells and red cell fragments	Mucin
Nuclear features	Mild-to-moderate atypia	Severe atypia
Mitoses	Occasional	Frequent
Stroma	Myxoid or hyalinized	Desmoplastic
Vascular invasion	Multicentric in large veins	Lymphovascular invasion around portal tracts

Angiosarcoma

Primary angiosarcomas are extremely rare, highly aggressive hepatic neoplasms. They have been historically associated with exposure to industrial toxins, vinyl chloride, arsenic compounds, and some types of contrast medium, namely Thorotrast [9, 11]. Angiosarcomas diffusely infiltrate the liver and most are not amenable to resection (Fig. 4.16). Liver transplantation is not effective in the management of patients with hepatic angiosarcoma because they develop recurrent disease in the graft at a median of 6 months and none survive more than 2 years [12, 13]. Hepatic angiosarcomas are composed of overtly malignant cells with enlarged, hyperchromatic nuclei, brisk mitotic activity, necrosis, and hemorrhage. The tumor cells grow along the pre-existing hepatic sinusoids and display nodular, papillary, or solid growth. Poorly-differentiated tumors contain epithelioid cells with abundant eosinophilic cytoplasm (Fig. 4.17).

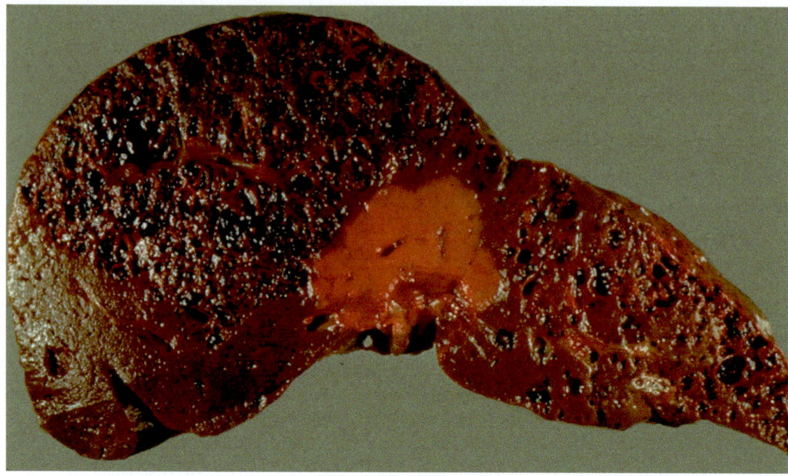

FIG. 4.16 Angiosarcomas contain dilated blood-filled vascular spaces that diffusely infiltrate the hepatic parenchyma.

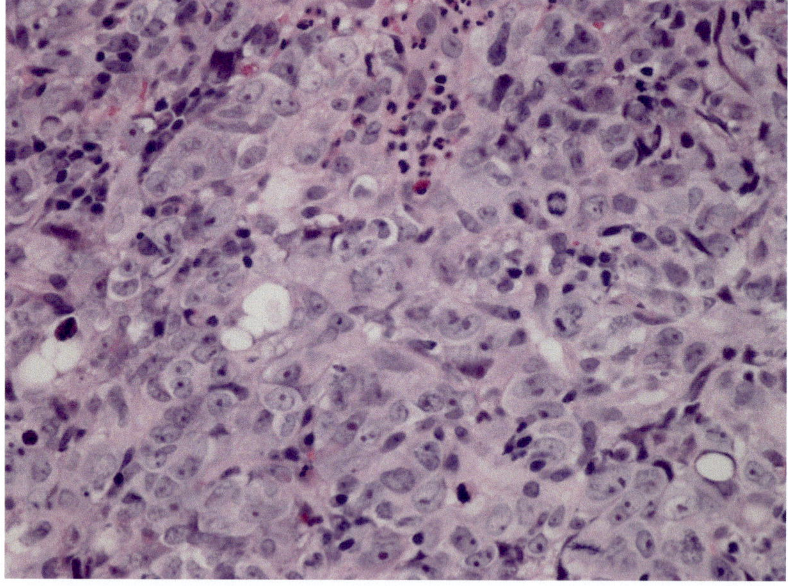

FIG. 4.17 Epithelioid angiosarcomas contain overtly malignant plump, round cells with large nuclei, and prominent nucleoli that simulate the features of carcinoma.

OTHER MESENCHYMAL NEOPLASMS

With the exceptions of the previously mentioned entities, other types of primary mesenchymal hepatic tumors are extremely rare (Table 4.3). Those that show smooth muscle differentiation are usually driven by Epstein–Barr virus (EBV) infection and occur among immunosuppressed patients with AIDS or solid organ transplants [14, 15]. These tumors consist of fascicles of smooth muscle cells admixed with primitive round cell areas and prominent intratumoral lymphocytes (Fig. 4.18). Inflammatory myofibroblastic tumors develop in patients of all ages, but are more common among children and young adults. They develop in multiple organs, including bladder, breast, pancreas, colon, and liver [16]. Although they have no metastatic potential, they are potentially locally aggressive and, thus, managed by resection [16]. Inflammatory myofibroblastic tumors are solitary, ill-defined lesions composed of whorled fascicles of spindle cells within fibrotic stroma (Fig. 4.19). They contain a mixed infiltrate of plasma cells, eosinophils, neutrophils, and lymphocytes (Fig. 4.20). Schwannomas rarely occur as primary hepatic neoplasms and are

TABLE 4.3 Spindle cell tumors of the liver.

Tumor	Histologic features	Patients affected
EBV-associated smooth muscle tumor	Spindle cells with eosinophilic cytoplasm	Immunosuppressed
	Primitive round cells	Adults > children
	Lymphocytes	
Schwannoma	Antoni A areas: densely cellular fascicles and nuclear palisading	Adults > children
	Antoni B areas: paucicellular, edematous	
	Tapered nuclei	
	Occasional bizarre hyperchromatic nuclei	
	Rare mitoses	
Gastrointestinal stromal tumor	Spindle or epithelioid cells	Adults > children
	Paranuclear vacuoles	
	Mild cytologic atypia despite high cellularity	
	Hyalinized stroma when treated	
Inflammatory myofibroblastic tumor	Plump spindle cells	Children > adults
	Plasma cell-predominant inflammatory infiltrate	

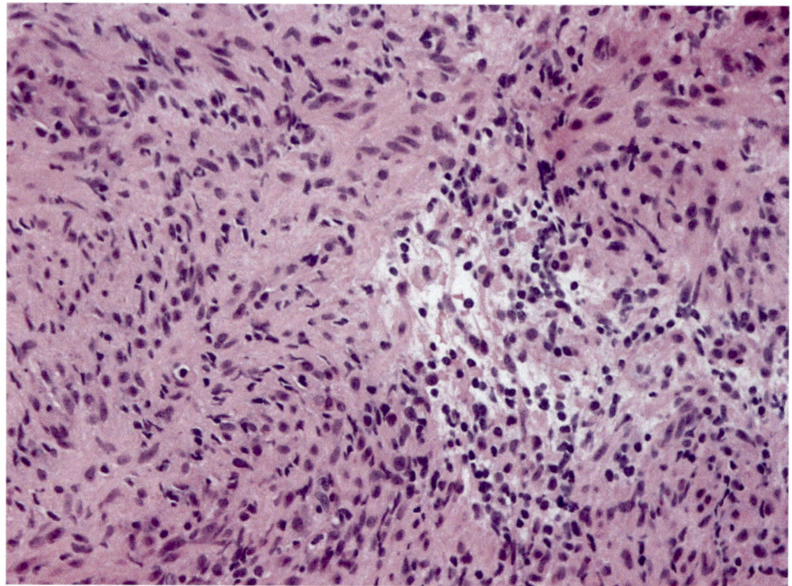

Fig. 4.18 An Epstein–Barr virus-associated smooth muscle tumor contains fascicles of smooth muscle cells admixed with round cells and scattered lymphocytes (photograph courtesy of Dr. Jinru Shia, Memorial Sloan-Kettering Cancer Center).

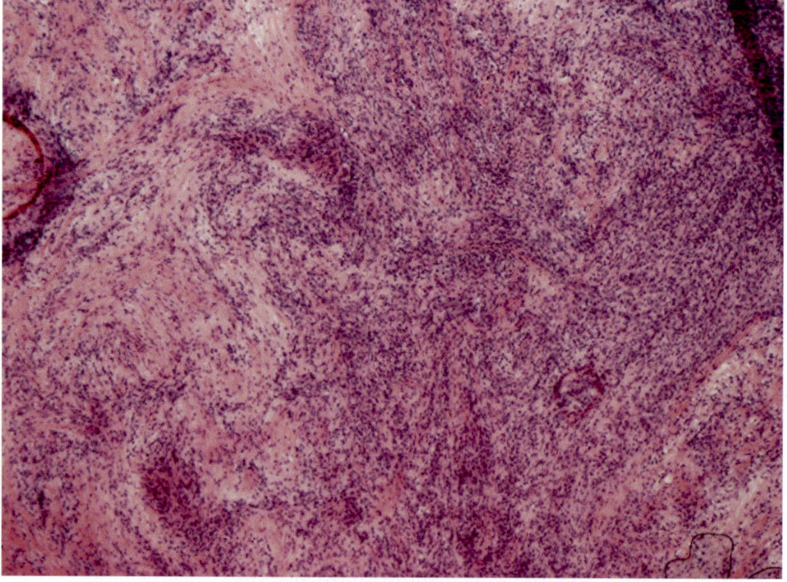

Fig. 4.19 The spindle cells of an inflammatory myofibroblastic tumor are arranged in interlacing fascicles.

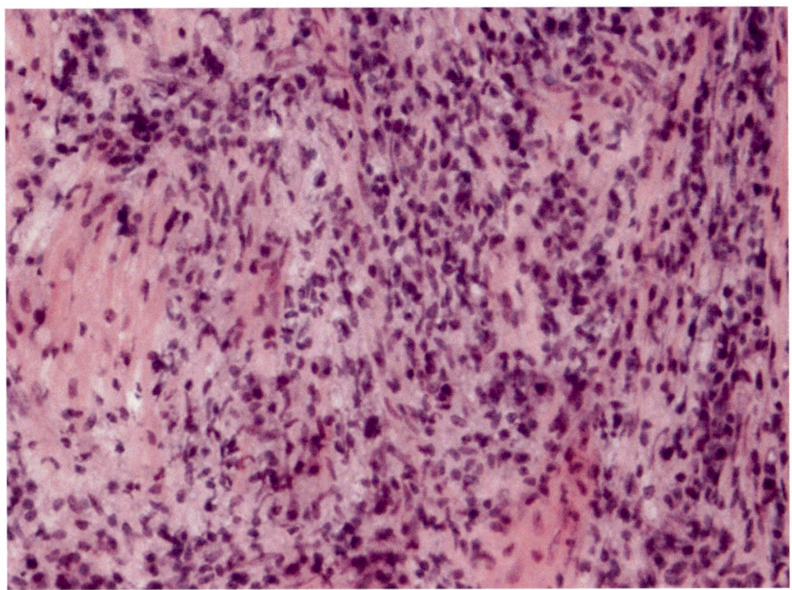

FIG. 4.20   The dense mixed inflammatory infiltrate of inflammatory myofibroblastic tumor obscures the tumor cells.

histologically similar to those that develop in soft tissues [17, 18]. They contain spindle cells with tapered faintly eosinophilic cytoplasm and elongated nuclei. One important entity to be considered in the differential diagnosis of hepatic mesenchymal neoplasms is primary, or metastatic, gastrointestinal stromal tumor. These lesions are usually quite cellular spindle cell tumors. Most are monomorphic and do not display appreciable mitotic activity or necrosis (Fig. 4.21). They are important to distinguish from other mesenchymal neoplasms because most are extremely susceptible to targeted chemotherapeutic agents. Tumors that have been preoperatively treated with a tyrosine kinase receptor inhibitor are paucicellular with striking stromal hyalinization [19].

PEDIATRIC MESENCHYMAL TUMORS
Hepatoblastoma
Hepatoblastomas occur sporadically and in association with both Beckwith-Wiedemann syndrome (gigantism, omphalocele, and macroglossia) and familial adenomatous polyposis [20, 21]. Patients are usually treated with a combination of chemotherapy and surgery, which can achieve 85–90% long-term disease-free survival rates [22–24].

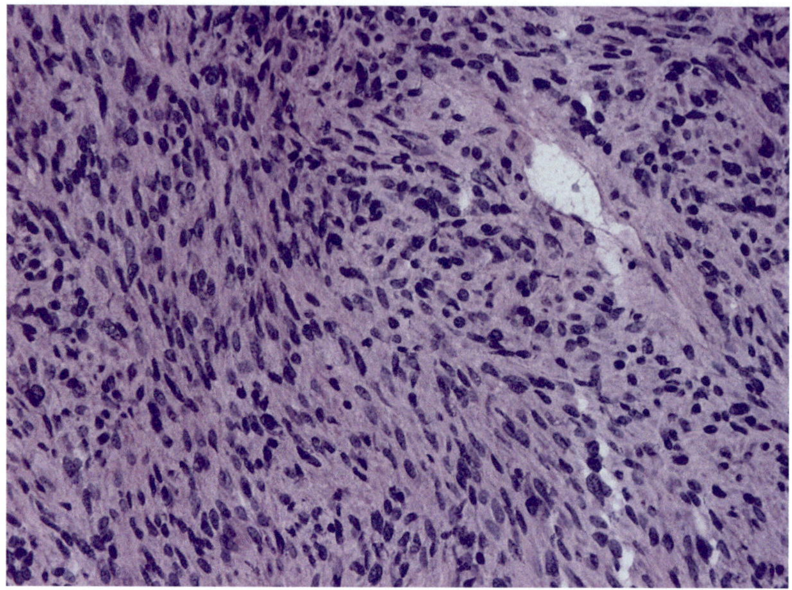

FIG. 4.21 Gastrointestinal stromal tumors contain spindle cells with abundant cytoplasm. Although quite cellular, they display minimal cytologic heterogeneity and mitotic figures are scarce.

Hepatoblastomas are large, multinodular masses with a heterogeneous cut surface, owing to hemorrhage and necrosis (Fig. 4.22). They may contain only epithelial elements, but most have mixed epithelial and mesenchymal components. The epithelial cells display a variety of histologic growth patterns and appearances, including embryonal, fetal, macrotrabecular, and anaplastic elements. Of these, embryonal and fetal patterns are most common. Tumors with an embryonal appearance contain small cells with round to ovoid nuclei and scant cytoplasm arranged in tubules, acini, or ribbon-like structures (Fig. 4.23). The fetal form resembles fetal liver, containing cells with a moderate amount of eosinophilic or clear cytoplasm and small, round nuclei (Fig. 4.24). Macrotrabecular hepatoblastoma closely resembles hepatocellular carcinoma and is composed of broad sheets of neoplastic cells with abundant eosinophilic cytoplasm (Fig. 4.25). Anaplastic tumors contain sheets of small round blue cells without hepatocellular differentiation and represent the most aggressive subtype of hepatoblastoma. Mesenchymal areas consist of primitive spindle cells in edematous stroma associated with osteoid (Fig. 4.26). Extramedullary hematopoiesis is often identified.

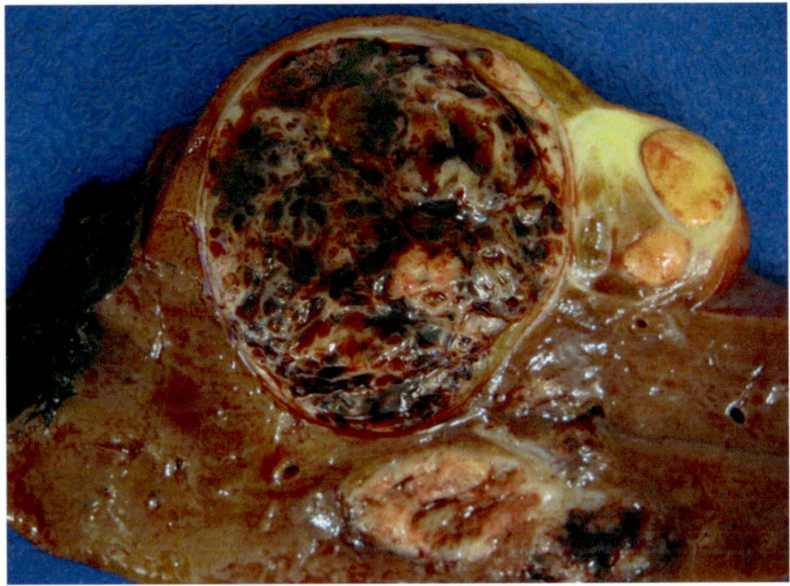

FIG. 4.22 This hepatoblastoma is pale yellow and brown with areas of hemorrhage (photograph courtesy of Dr. Debra Beneck, Weill Cornell Medical College).

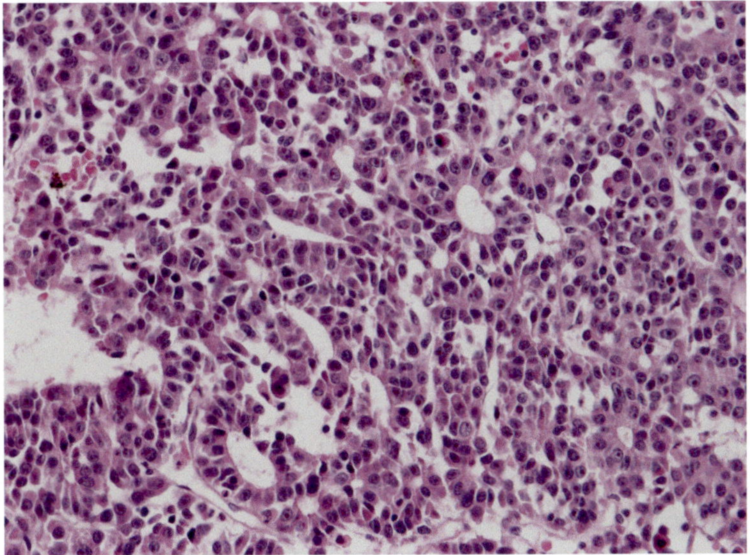

FIG. 4.23 The embryonal pattern of hepatoblastoma displays cells with round nuclei and eosinophilic cytoplasm arranged in ribbons and gland-like structures (photograph courtesy of Dr. Debra Beneck, Weill Cornell Medical College).

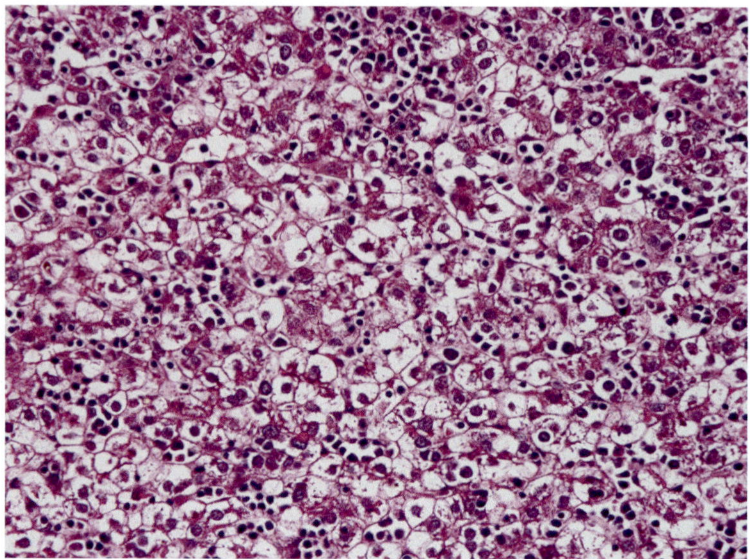

FIG. 4.24 Round cells with clear cytoplasm and small nuclei are typical of the fetal pattern of hepatoblastoma (photograph courtesy of Dr. Debra Beneck, Weill Cornell Medical College).

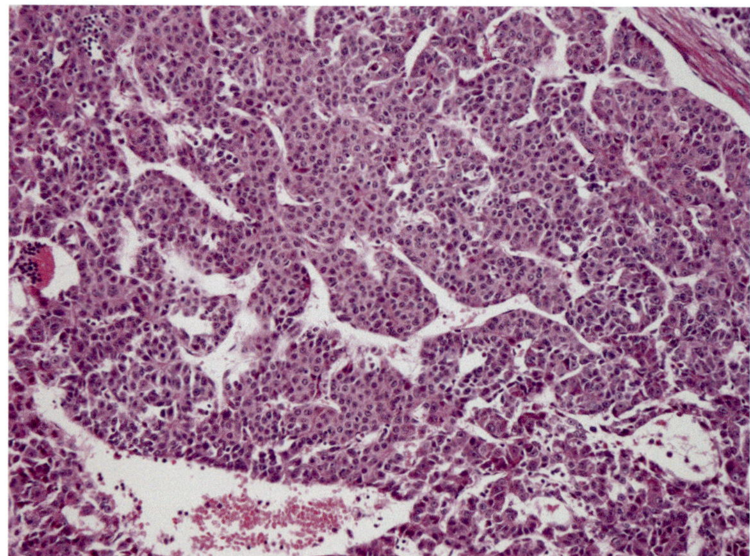

FIG. 4.25 The macrotrabecular pattern of hepatoblastoma resembles hepatocellular carcinoma. Trabeculae of tumor cells are separated by dilated sinusoidal spaces (photograph courtesy of Dr. Debra Beneck, Weill Cornell Medical College).

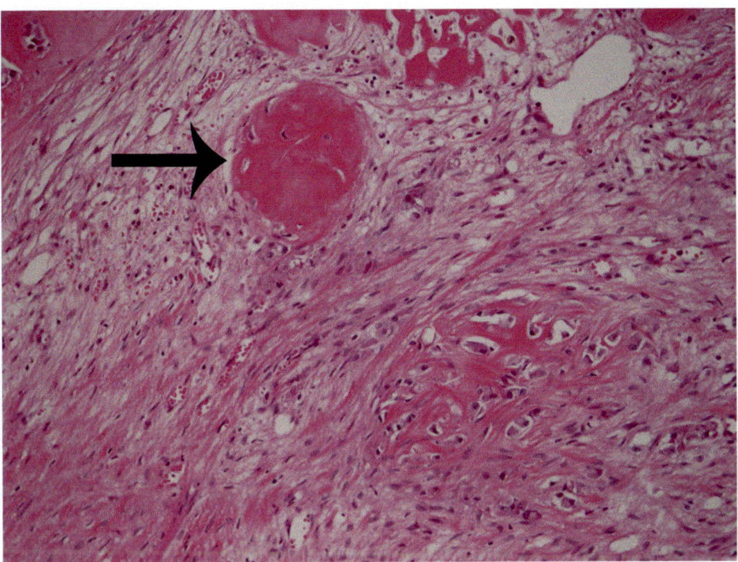

FIG. 4.26 Hepatoblastomas with mesenchymal elements contain primitive spindle cells and deposits of osteoid (*arrow*) (photograph courtesy of Dr. Debra Beneck, Weill Cornell Medical College).

Infantile Hemangioendothelioma

Infantile hemangioendothelioma is the most common purely mesenchymal liver tumor of pediatric patients. These lesions may cause cardiac failure due to their large size and/or multifocality, so they are typically resected despite their benign nature. Infantile hemangioendotheliomas are solitary or, more frequently, multifocal, poorly circumscribed, hemorrhagic tumors with solid and cystic areas (Fig. 4.27). They contain variably sized, irregular vascular channels lined by a single layer of endothelial cells within edematous stroma. Most tumor cells contain bland nuclei without appreciable mitotic activity, although slight nuclear enlargement and hyperchromasia may be seen in some cases (Fig. 4.28).

Mesenchymal Hamartoma

Mesenchymal hamartomas are benign solitary tumors that are more commonly detected in pediatric patients, but they may rarely come to clinical attention in adult patients. They are ill-defined, variegated solid and cystic tumors with variable amounts of fibrosis that imparts a myxoid appearance (Fig. 4.29). Mesenchymal hamartomas are composed of disorganized nodules of normal-appearing

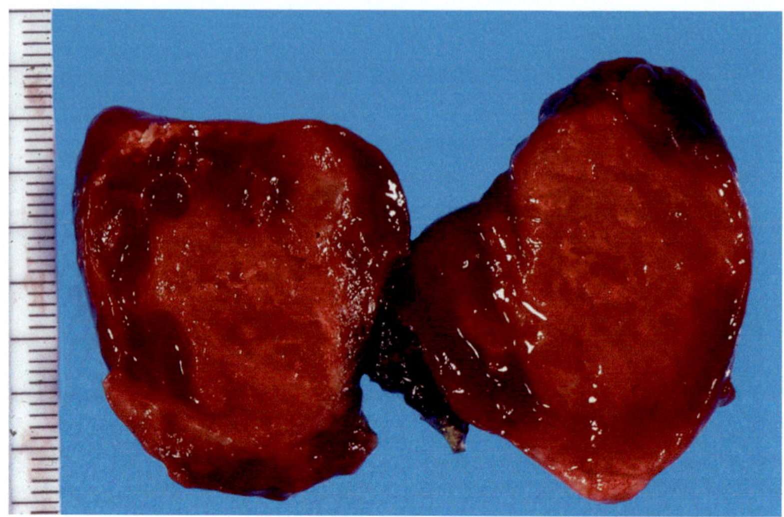

FIG. 4.27 Infantile hemangioendotheliomas are unencapsulated, spongy, hemorrhagic tumors (photograph courtesy of Dr. Debra Beneck, Weill Cornell Medical College).

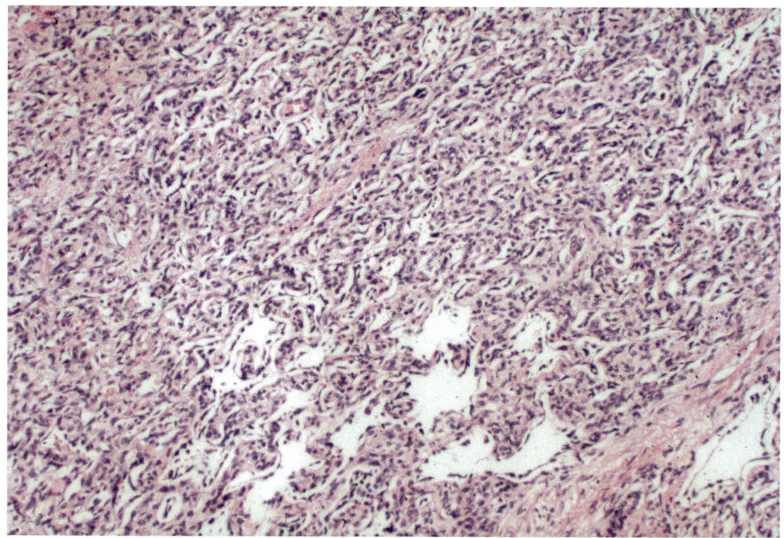

FIG. 4.28 Irregular vascular spaces are separated by loose mesenchymal tissue in an infantile hemangioendothelioma. The tumor is quite cellular, but cytologically bland without necrosis (photograph courtesy of Dr. Debra Beneck, Weill Cornell Medical College).

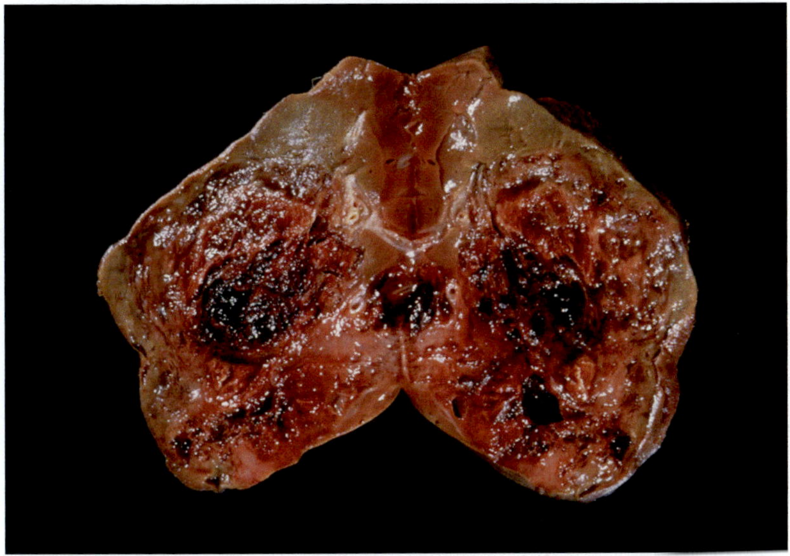

FIG. 4.29 This mesenchymal hamartoma has a heterogeneous solid and cystic cut surface with hemorrhage.

hepatocytes and proliferating bile ducts within loose fibrous stroma (Figs. 4.30 and 4.31). Ectatic vascular spaces and cysts lined by flattened cuboidal epithelium are present in fibrotic areas (Figs. 4.31 and 4.32). Extramedullary hematopoiesis may be identified as well.

Undifferentiated Embryonal Sarcoma

Undifferentiated embryonal sarcoma is a rare pediatric tumor that pursues an aggressive clinical course. Surgical resection offers the best opportunity for cure, although patients with bilobar hepatic disease are not resectable, or may be considered for liver transplantation [25]. Undifferentiated embryonal sarcomas are large, bulky tumors composed of spindle and stellate cells within myxoid stroma (Fig. 4.33). These tumor cells contain abundant bubbly cytoplasm and PAS-positive, diastase-resistant eosinophilic globules (Fig. 4.34). Mitotic figures are numerous and extramedullary hematopoiesis is usually present.

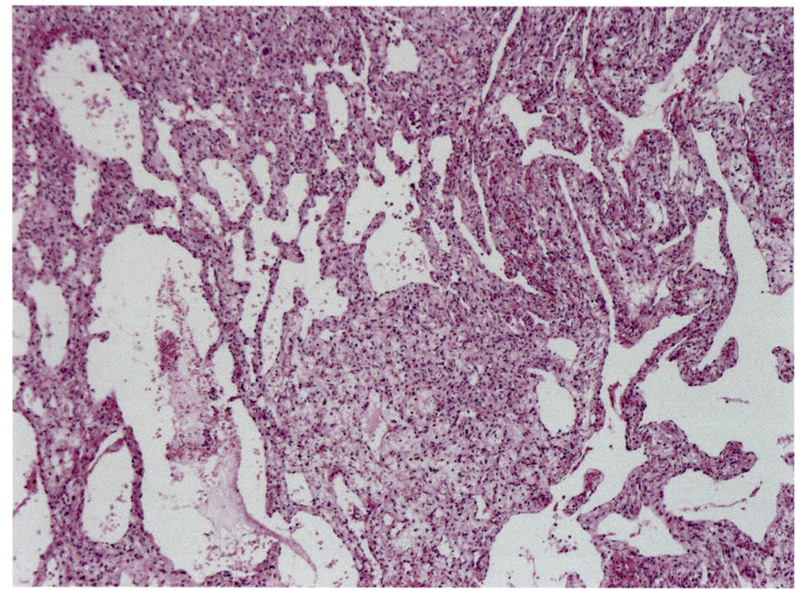

FIG. 4.30 Mesenchymal hamartomas contain normal hepatic elements, including aggregates of hepatocytes, cystic spaces, and loose stroma.

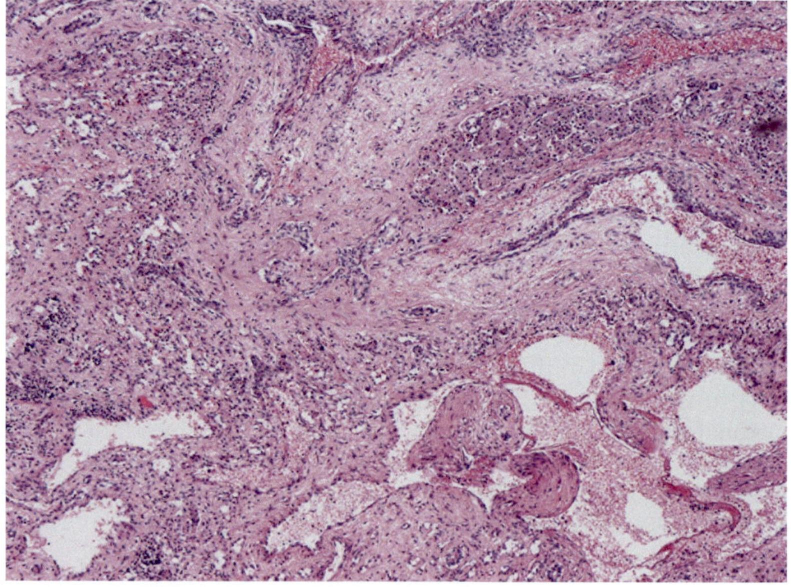

FIG. 4.31 Mesenchymal hamartomas also contain fibrotic areas with proliferating ductules and ectatic blood vessels.

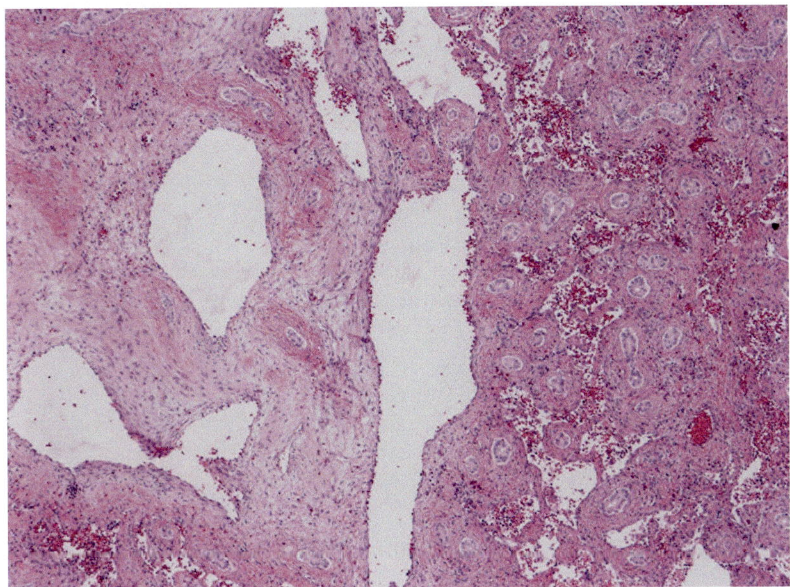

FIG. 4.32 Cysts of mesenchymal hamartomas are lined by cuboidal or flat epithelium.

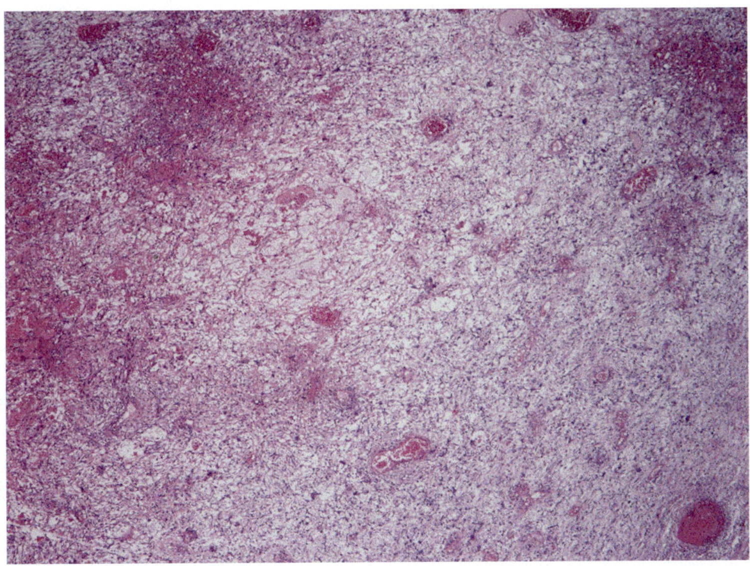

FIG. 4.33 Undifferentiated embryonal sarcomas are malignant tumors composed of a disorganized proliferation of spindle cells in hemorrhagic, myxoid stroma.

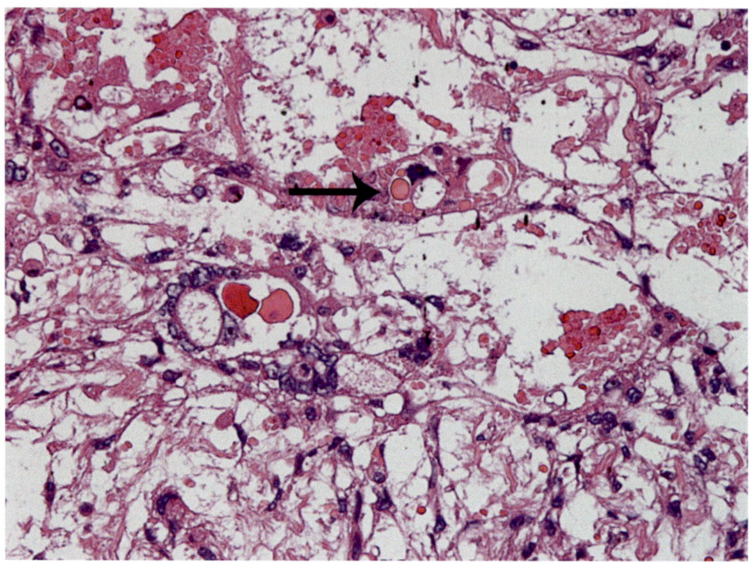

Fig. 4.34 The cells of undifferentiated embryonal sarcoma are primitive-appearing spindle and stellate cells. Some contain intracytoplasmic hyaline globules (*arrow*).

References

1. Flemming P, Lang H, Georgii A. Mesenchymal tumors of the liver: their frequency and histopathologic diagnostic problems in surgical investigations. Verh Dtsch Ges Pathol. 1995;79:116–9.
2. Hornick JL, Fletcher CD. PEComa: what do we know so far? Histopathology. 2006;48(1):75–82.
3. Rouquie D, Eggenspieler P, Algayres JP, Bechade D, Camparo P, Baranger B. Malignant-like angiomyolipoma of the liver: report of one case and review of the literature. Ann Chir. 2006;131(5):338–41.
4. Bioulac-Sage P, Laumonier H, Laurent C, Blanc JF, Balabaud C. Benign and malignant vascular tumors of the liver in adults. Semin Liver Dis. 2008;28(3):302–14.
5. Kim T, Hori M, Onishi H. Liver masses with a central or eccentric scar. Semin Ultrasound CT MR. 2009;30(5):418–25.
6. Mosoia L, Mabrut J-Y, Adham M, et al. Hepatic epithelioid hemangioendothelioma: long-term results of surgical management. J Surg Oncol. 2008;98:432–7.
7. Ercolani G, Grazi GL, Pinna AD. Liver transplantation for benign hepatic tumors: a systematic review. Dig Surg. 2010;27(1):68–75.
8. Mehrabi A, Kashfi A, Fonouni H, et al. Primary malignant hepatic epithelioid hemangioendothelioma: a comprehensive review of the literature with emphasis on the surgical therapy. Cancer. 2006;107(9):2108–21.
9. Bonaccorsi-Riani E, Lerut JP. Liver transplantation and vascular tumors. Transpl Int. 2010;23(7):686–91.

10. Weiss SW, Enzinger FM. Epithelioid hemangioendothelioma: a vascular tumor often mistaken for a carcinoma. Cancer. 1982;50(5):970–81.
11. Bolt HM. Vinyl chloride-a classical industrial toxicant of new interest. Crit Rev Toxicol. 2005;35(4):307–23.
12. Husted TL, Neff G, Thomas MJ, Gross TG, Woodle ES, Buell JF. Liver transplantation for primary or metastatic sarcoma to the liver. Am J Transplant. 2006;6:392–7.
13. Weitz J, Klimstra DS, Cymes K, et al. Management of primary liver sarcomas. Cancer. 2007;109(7):1391–6.
14. Deyrup AT. Epstein-Barr virus-associated epithelial and mesenchymal neoplasms. Hum Pathol. 2008;39(4):473–83.
15. Cheuk W, Li PC, Chan JK. Epstein-Barr virus-associated smooth muscle tumour: a distinctive mesenchymal tumour of immunocompromised individuals. Pathology. 2002;34(3):245–9.
16. Kovach SJ, Fischer AC, Katzman PJ, et al. Inflammatory myofibroblastic tumors. J Surg Oncol. 2006;94(5):385–91.
17. Ozkan EE, Gulder ME, Uzunkoy A. A case report of benign schwannoma of the liver. Intern Med. 2010;49(15):1533–6.
18. Lee WH, Kim TH, You SS, et al. Benign schwannoma of the liver: a case report. J Korean Med Sci. 2008;23(4):727–30.
19. Mushtaq S, Mamoon N, Hassan U, Iqbal M, Khadim MT, Sarfraz T. Gastrointestinal stromal tumors-a morphologic and immunohistochemical study. J Gastrointest Cancer. 2009;40:109–14.
20. Garber JE, Li FP, Kingston JE, et al. Hepatoblastoma and familial adenomatous polyposis. J Natl Cancer Inst. 1988;80(20):1626–8.
21. Hughes LJ, Michels VV. Risk of hepatoblastoma in familial adenomatous polyposis. Am J Med Genet. 1992;43(6):1023–5.
22. Fuchs J, Rydzynski J, von Schweinitz D, et al. Pretreatment prognostic factors and treatment results in childhood hepatoblastoma: a report from the German Cooperative Pediatric Liver Tumor Study HB 94. Cancer. 2002;95(1):172–82.
23. Pritchard J, Stringer M. Outcome and complications after resection of hepatoblastoma. J Pediatr Surg. 2004;39(11):1743–4.
24. Czauderna P, Otto JB, Roebuck DJ, von Schweinitz D, Plaschkes J. Surgical treatment of hepatoblastoma in children. Pediatr Radiol. 2006;36(3):187–91.
25. Kelly M, Martin L, Alonso M, Altura R. Liver transplant for relapsed undifferentiated embryonal sarcoma in a young child. J Pediatr Surg. 2009;44(12):e1–3.

Chapter 5
Intraoperative Assessment of Donor Livers in the Transplant Setting

INTRODUCTION

Solid organ transplants are increasingly performed at specialized centers across the country and more hospitals are accredited to perform these surgeries each year. Clinical features such as donor age >60 years, cold ischemic time >12 h, donation after cardiac death, prolonged stay in the intensive care unit, and history of malignancy are relative contraindications to liver donation [1]. Unfortunately, one factor that limits the number of successful liver transplant procedures is the shortage of available donor organs. Thus, some centers have resorted to living-related donors and extended donor programs to address patient needs. Deceased-donor extended criteria include donor age >65 years, donation after cardiac death, positive viral serology (hepatitis C or hepatitis B core antibody), prior history of malignancy, steatosis, and high-risk behaviors [1]. Living-related donors routinely undergo preoperative radiographic evaluation of the liver and its vasculature, but abdominal imaging studies from deceased donors are not always available. For this reason, nodules in cadaveric livers are often first identified during organ harvest or transplantation. These lesions are usually submitted for intraoperative frozen section evaluation in order to determine whether the liver is suitable for transplantation. Biopsies are also obtained from the donor liver for two major indications: to evaluate for the presence and extent of steatosis and to assess extent of fibrosis in patients with underlying liver disease.

95

R.K. Yantiss (ed.), *Frozen Section Library: Liver, Extrahepatic Biliary Tree and Gallbladder*, Frozen Section Library, DOI 10.1007/978-1-4614-0043-1_5,
© Springer Science+Business Media, LLC 2011

INCIDENTALLY DISCOVERED LIVER LESIONS

Small benign tumors, such as bile duct adenomas, bile duct hamartomas, and sclerotic hemangiomas, are frequently encountered in donor livers and may be submitted for frozen section analysis during organ harvest or at the time of liver transplantation. The histologic features of these entities are discussed in detail in Chapters 2 and 4. Hepatocellular adenomas and focal nodular hyperplasia may also occur in donor organs from young women as discussed in Chapter 1. Malignant primary hepatic tumors are not a diagnostic consideration in most donor livers since they develop in patients with advanced liver disease that prohibits use of the organ as a graft. The pathologic features of incidental primary hepatic tumors encountered in donor livers are enumerated in Table 5.1.

Donor transmission of malignant tumors *via* solid organ transplantation is exceedingly rare, occurring in only 0.02–0.2% of patients [2]. Most malignancies that are transmitted to the recipient in this fashion become manifest within 1 year of transplantation and presumably result from micrometastases, or circulating tumor cells, present in the graft at the time of harvest [3]. Malignant melanoma is the most common transmitted malignancy and accounts for 28% of all cases, followed in frequency by non–small-cell lung cancer, renal cell carcinoma, choriocarcinoma, and high-grade gliomas [3–6]. The presence of a malignancy in the donor is usually unsuspected at the time of harvest, although transmission of gliomas in donor organs is so uncommon that patients with known brain tumors are not excluded from organ donation. Discovery of a donor-transmitted malignancy is a catastrophic event that requires cessation of immunosuppressive therapy and emergent retransplantation, and thus, most surgeons have a low threshold for biopsy of incidentally discovered nodules during organ harvest [7].

STEATOSIS

Donor livers are routinely evaluated for the presence of macrovesicular steatosis, which is considered the most important histologic feature predictive of immediate graft function. Fat accumulation in hepatocytes leads to increased cell volume, which impedes perfusion of hepatic parenchyma. Steatosis also impairs mitochondrial function, such that fatty hepatocytes have diminished capacity for restoration of ATP levels following reperfusion [8, 9]. Data from several studies suggest that donor livers with mild macrovesicular steatosis (<30% of hepatocytes) in liver biopsy samples function similarly to nonfatty livers in the perioperative period, whereas postoperative complications and graft failure are more common in livers with macrovesicular steatosis in >30% of hepatocytes (Figs. 5.1 and 5.2)

TABLE 5.1   Incidental primary hepatic tumors in donor livers.

Tumor	Gross features	Histologic features
Bile duct adenoma	Solitary or multiple white nodules Frequently subcapsular	Well circumscribed Tightly packed monotonous small tubules in cellular stroma Low cuboidal epithelium Round, basally located nuclei Occasional luminal mucin
Bile duct hamartoma	Solitary or multiple white nodules Frequently subcapsular Multiple tumors near portal tracts	Well circumscribed Evenly spaced tubules in collagenous stroma Variably dilated tubules Flattened or cuboidal epithelium Luminal bile or inspissated proteinaceous material
Sclerotic hemangioma	Gray–white nodule Frequently subcapsular	Compressed vascular spaces Flat endothelial cells Abundant hyalinized stroma
Hepatocellular adenoma	Pale brown or yellow May be hemorrhagic Frequently subcapsular	Sheets of normal-appearing hepatocytes Thick cell plates Fibrous septa, but no portal tracts Solitary parenchymal arteries
Focal nodular hyperplasia	Round pale brown tumor Prominent fibrous septa or central scar	Normal hepatocytes separated by radiating septa Bile ductular proliferation along septal margins Thick-walled arteries within septa

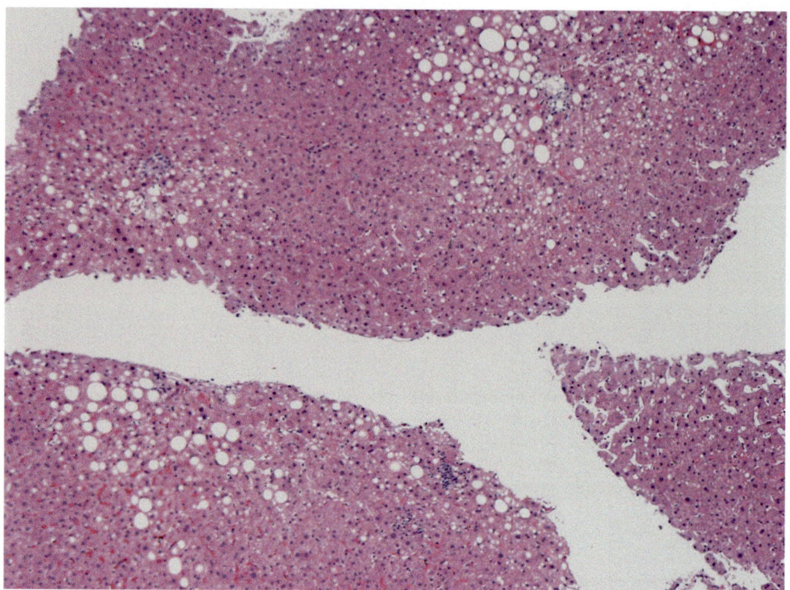

FIG. 5.1 Approximately 5–10% of hepatocytes show fat accumulation in this liver needle biopsy sample. Inflammatory activity is negligible.

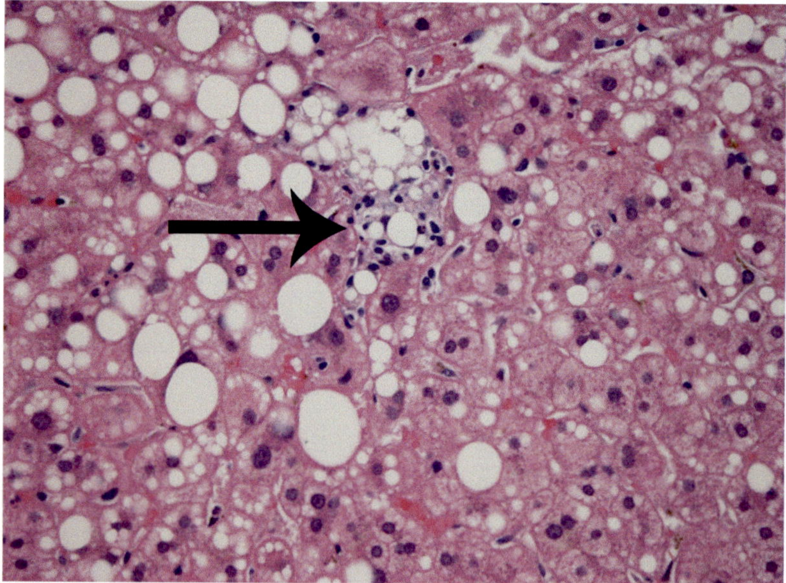

FIG. 5.2 Large cytoplasmic fat vacuoles compress and displace hepatocyte nuclei. A single inflammatory focus is present (*arrow*).

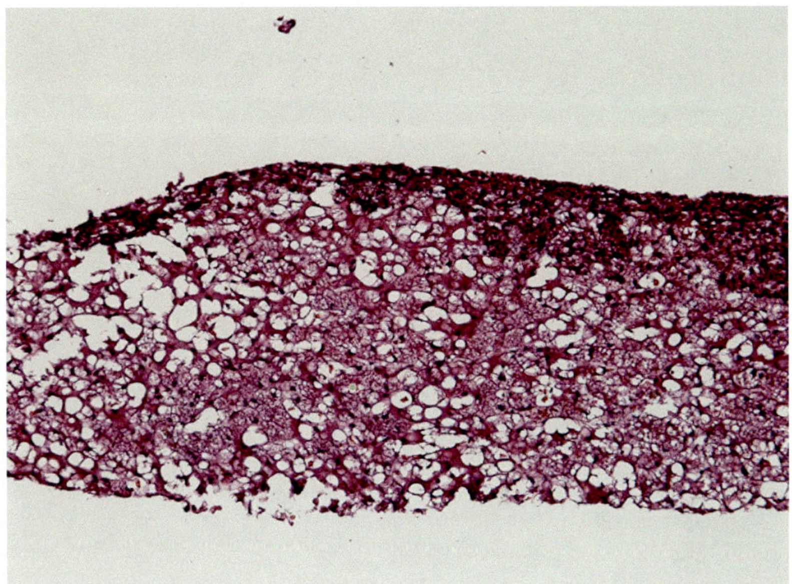

Fig. 5.3 Approximately 40% of hepatocytes in this donor liver biopsy show macrovesicular steatosis. Fatty hepatocytes contain vacuoles that distend the cells.

[1, 10, 11]. Livers that contain fat in 30–50% of hepatocytes may not function well in the perioperative period, but most patients who receive grafts with this amount of steatosis have a favorable outcome following transplantation, particularly if they have good performance status and no co-morbid disease. However, steatosis in >60% of hepatocytes is associated with high rates of graft failure and increased risk of death [12–14]. Thus, donor livers that show steatosis in <30% of hepatocytes are routinely used for transplantation and those with 30–60% steatosis are also accepted for transplantation in most patients (Figs. 5.3 and 5.4). Donor livers with steatosis affecting >60% of hepatocytes are at substantial risk of graft failure, so their use is limited to emergency situations or as a bridge until a more suitable graft becomes available (Figs. 5.5 and 5.6). Steatotic donor livers are enlarged and pale, so the surgeon is alerted to the possibility of excess fat and prompted to obtain an intraoperative frozen section. Liver biopsy with frozen section evaluation is considered the gold standard for assessing extent of steatosis in donor livers, although overestimation of steatosis is a relatively common problem because fatty hepatocytes are much larger than those without cytoplasmic fat [15].

Microvesicular steatosis is seen in donor liver biopsies from patients with obesity, sepsis, and traumatic death (Fig. 5.7) [10].

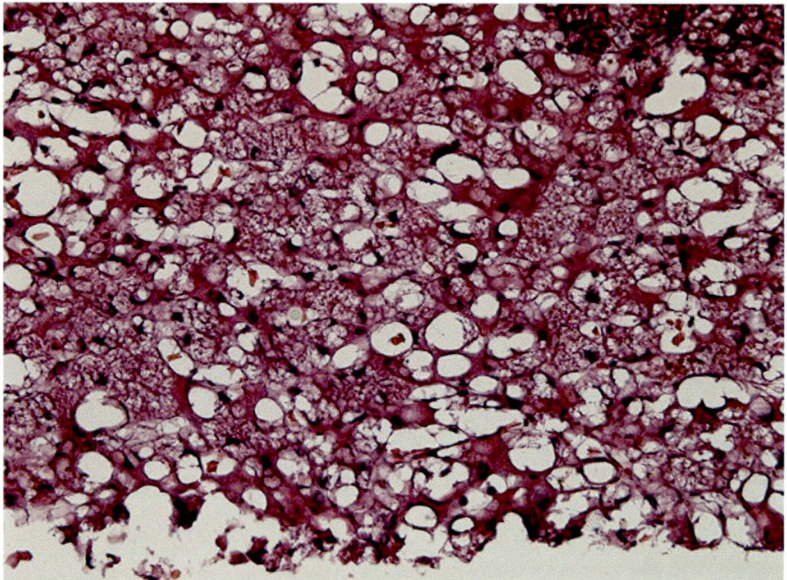

FIG. 5.4 Steatotic hepatocytes comprise approximately 40% of volume of this biopsy specimen. The background liver cells contain rarified cytoplasm, which represents a freezing artifact.

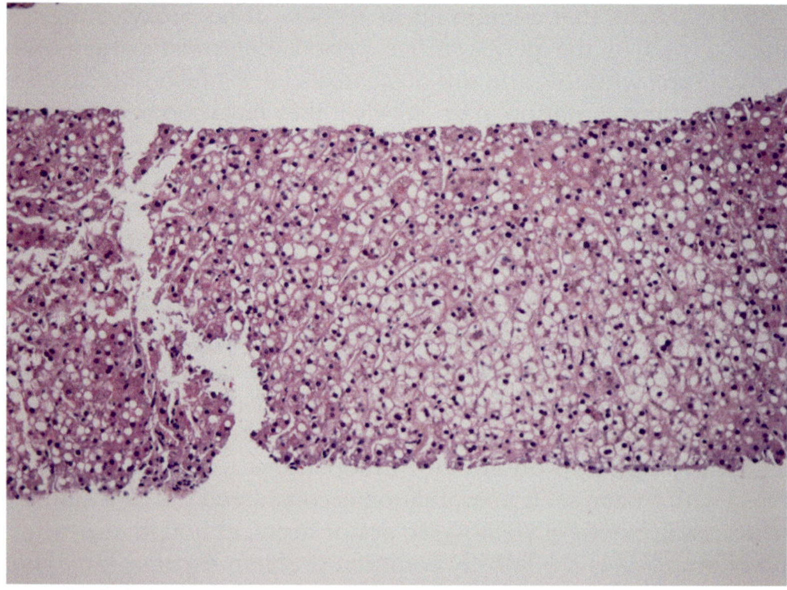

FIG. 5.5 Approximately 70% of hepatocytes contain fat vacuoles. Inflammation is minimal.

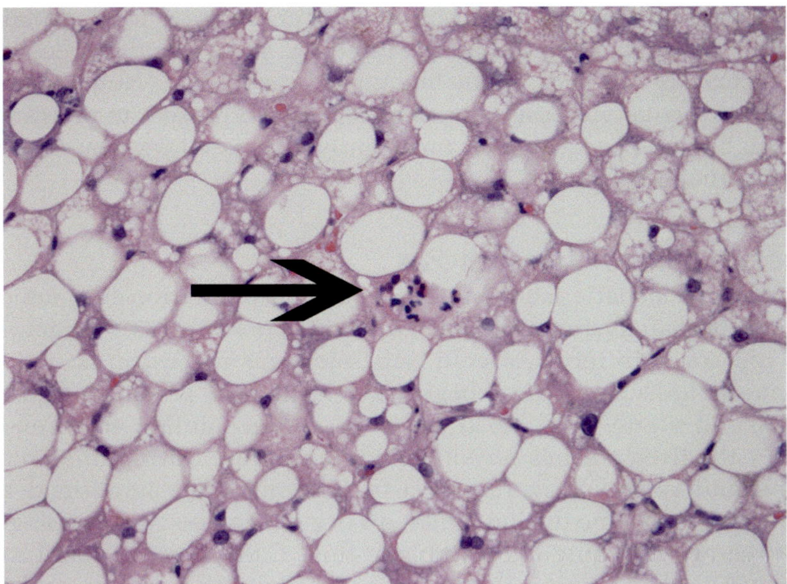

FIG. 5.6 Predominantly macrovesicular steatosis is present in approximately 80% of hepatocytes. A focus of neutrophilic inflammation is present in the lobule (*arrow*).

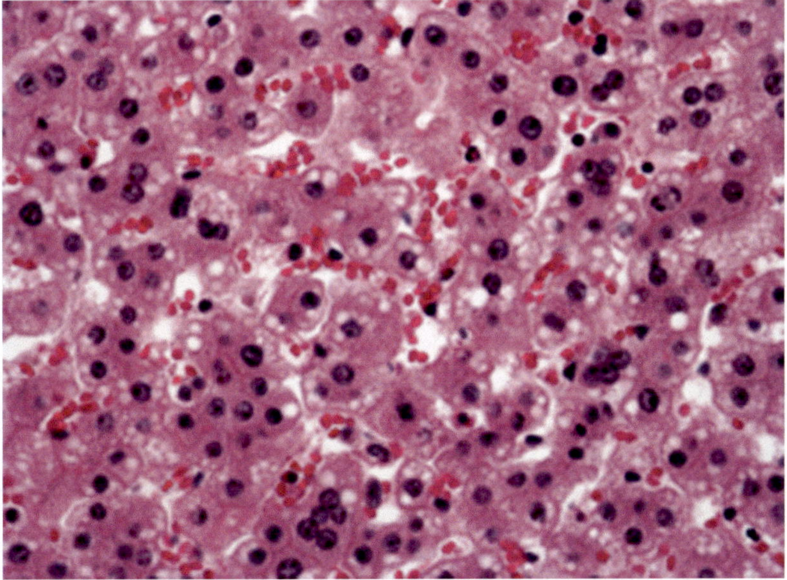

FIG. 5.7 Microvesicular steatosis appears as multiple tiny vacuoles within the hepatocyte cytoplasm.

It is not regarded as an absolute contraindication to transplantation or risk factor for poor long-term graft function because it generally resolves following engraftment [10]. Nonetheless, microvesicular steatosis should be reported if present in pretransplant biopsies because it is consistently associated with early poor graft function [16].

HEPATOCELLULAR NECROSIS

Prolonged hepatic ischemia prior to transplantation is a major cause of graft dysfunction. The duration of pretransplant ischemia is measured in terms of cold ischemic time and warm ischemic time. Cold ischemic time begins when the liver is removed from its blood supply and cooled with a perfusion solution and it ends after the liver reaches physiologic temperature during implantation and revascularization. Warm ischemic time is defined as the period of time during which an organ remains at physiologic temperature despite reduced blood flow. Cold ischemia that lasts longer than 12 hours promotes hepatocellular necrosis and is associated with poor graft function [17]. Livers procured following cardiac death are often subjected to a prolonged warm ischemic interval that promotes cell death, so these organs are classified under extended donor criteria. They tend to be used only at major transplant centers where surgeons may request frozen section analysis to evaluate the extent of hepatocellular injury [18]. Livers subjected to prolonged warm ischemia show a variable degree of hepatocyte necrosis that is most pronounced around central veins and progresses toward the portal tracts (Fig. 5.8). Hepatocellular necrosis affecting more than 10% of the parenchyma is associated with graft nonfunction, so these livers are generally discarded [19–21]. Important points for pathologists to note in their frozen section diagnoses include a percentage estimate of hepatocyte necrosis, as well as any amount of steatosis and inflammation.

DONOR LIVERS FROM PATIENTS WITH CHRONIC HEPATITIS C VIRAL INFECTION

Livers from patients with positive HCV serologies may be transplanted into recipients with HCV-induced HCC or decompensated cirrhosis [22]. These organs are considered acceptable for transplantation according to extended donor criteria, provided they show only mild inflammatory activity and fibrosis [23]. Biopsy of the donor liver may be obtained prior to transplantation in order

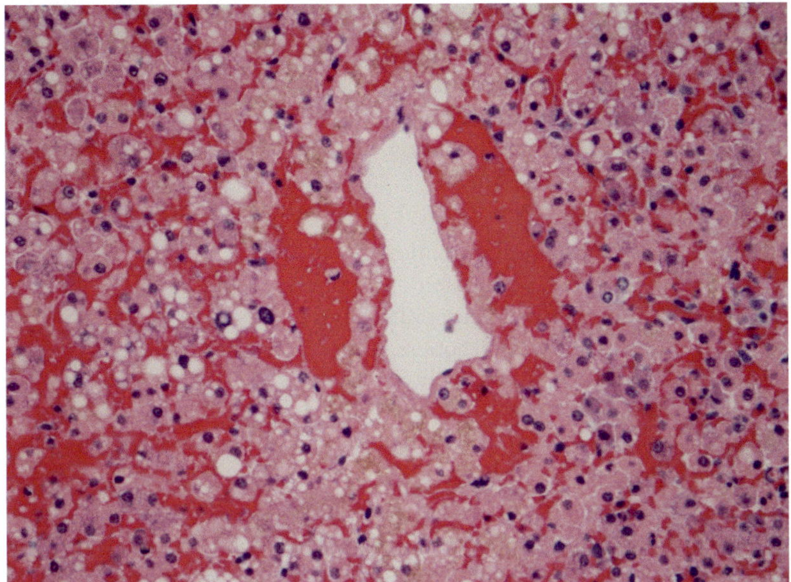

FIG. 5.8 Prolonged warm ischemic time promotes centrilobular necrosis accompanied by hemorrhage. This graft failed immediately after transplantation.

to determine the severity of inflammatory activity and extent of fibrosis (Table 5.2). Portal inflammation without interface hepatitis, or only limited interface hepatitis (grade 2/4 or less), does not preclude use of the graft. Moderately active hepatitis with easily detectable interface hepatitis and lobular injury predicts poor overall graft survival and a high risk of severe HCV-related chronic hepatitis following transplantation (Figs. 5.9–5.11). Early fibrous expansion of portal tracts is not always appreciable at the time of frozen section, but this finding is not a contraindication to transplantation (Fig. 5.12). Donor livers that show bridging fibrosis or nodule formation, however, are generally considered unacceptable for transplantation and discarded (Figs. 5.13 and 5.14). Precise classification of disease severity at frozen section is not necessary, but pathologists should note whether inflammatory activity and fibrosis exceed grade 2/4 and stage 2/4, respectively, since mild disease does not preclude transplantation of HCV-positive livers into HCV-infected patients.

TABLE 5.2 Grading and staging of chronic viral hepatitis.

	Description
Portal activity grade	
0	No or minimal inflammation
1	Portal inflammation only
2	Mild interface hepatitis
3	Moderate interface hepatitis
4	Severe interface hepatitis
Lobular activity grade	
0	No or minimal inflammation
1	Inflammation, but no acidophil bodies
2	Inflammation and acidophil bodies
3	Inflammation with frequent acidophil bodies or confluent necrosis without bridging
4	Bridging necrosis
Fibrosis stage	
0	No or minimal fibrosis
1	Fibrous expansion of portal tracts
2	Periportal or portal–portal fibrous septa with intact architecture
3	Bridging fibrosis with architectural distortion and nodule formation
4	Cirrhosis

Based on data from: Scheuer [29]

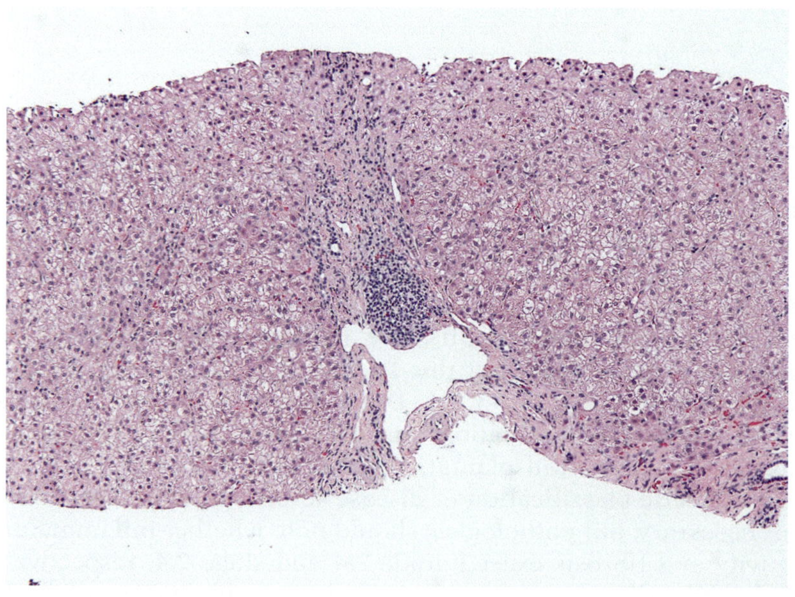

FIG. 5.9 Chronic, mildly active HCV-related hepatitis produces rounded lymphoid aggregates in portal tracts without appreciable lobular injury.

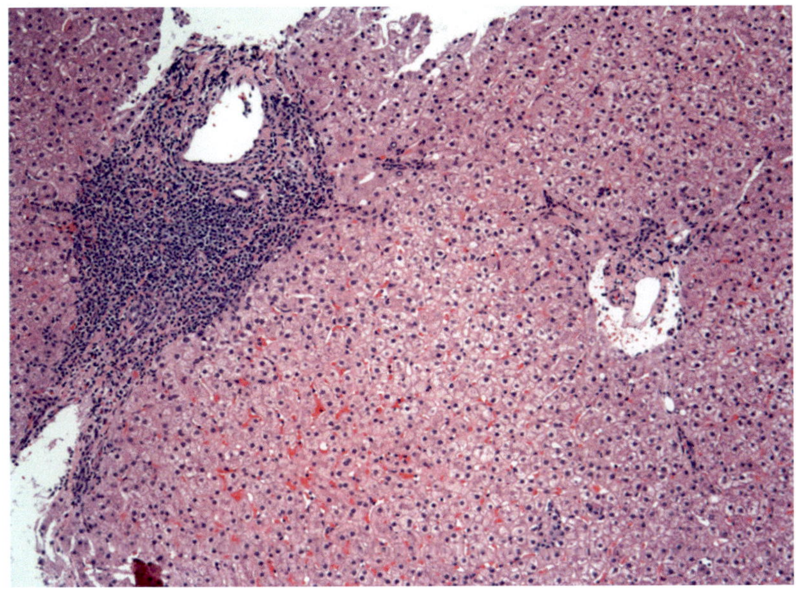

FIG. 5.10 Lymphoid aggregates in mild HCV-related chronic hepatitis are smooth and limited to the fibrous tissue of a portal tract.

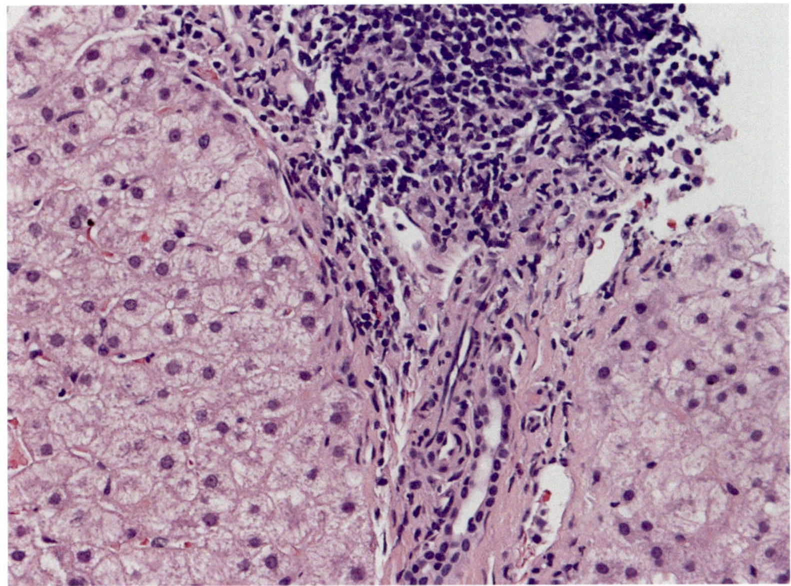

FIG. 5.11 Early HCV-related hepatic fibrosis is centered on portal tracts. This portal tract is fibrotic and expanded, but bridging fibrosis is lacking.

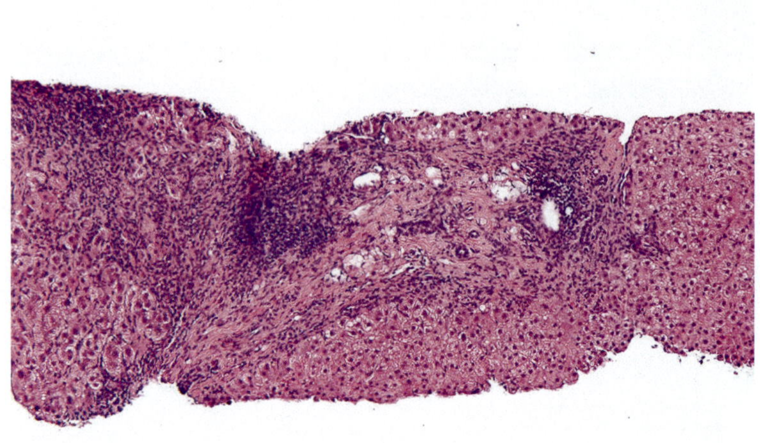

FIG. 5.12 Advanced HCV-related disease is evidenced by the presence of multiple lymphoid aggregates. The liver core has an irregular contour, which reflects the presence of fibrous bridges.

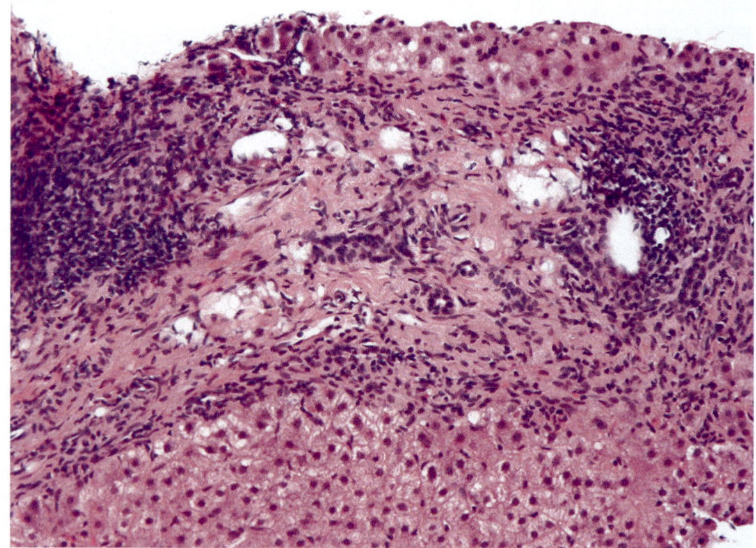

FIG. 5.13 Advanced HCV-related disease is characterized by bridging fibrosis with broad fibrous septa with dense lymphoid aggregates and proliferating ductules. A liver with this degree of fibrosis and inflammation is not suitable for transplantation.

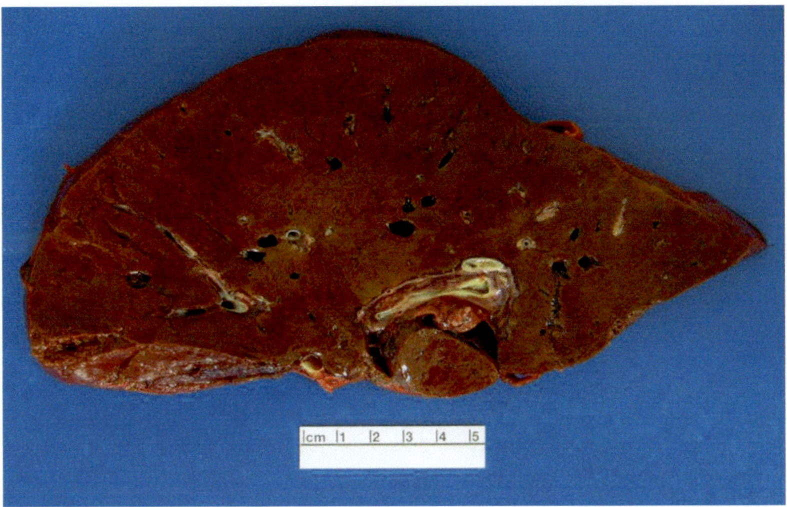

FIG. 5.14 This liver failed during transplant surgery and was immediately removed. The liver was swollen with a ruptured capsule. The cut surface has a mottled appearance.

PRIMARY ALLOGRAFT NONFUNCTION

Up to 10% of donor livers never function properly in the posttransplant period and rare allografts fail intraoperatively (Figs. 5.14 and 5.15) [24]. The term "primary graft nonfunction" has been used to describe transplanted organs that function poorly in the immediate posttransplant period. Factors that have been implicated in development of graft nonfunction include discrepant donor-to-recipient weight ratios, low preoperative platelet counts, prolonged duration of surgery, and selection of organ preservation solution; but most cases are attributed to preservation/reperfusion injury [25, 26]. The precise mechanisms of injury are unclear, but prolonged cold and warm ischemic times promote death of sinusoidal endothelial cells and hepatocytes. Injured and necrotic cells induce hypercoagulability, aggregation of inflammatory cells and platelets, and compromise of microcirculation in the hepatic parenchyma. Propagation of injury secondarily damages more hepatocytes and produces massive necrosis within a few hours of transplantation (Figs. 5.16 and 5.17) [27].

The histologic features of nonfunctional grafts are variable. Early histologic changes associated with preservation/reperfusion injury include hepatocyte ballooning and necrosis with vacuolization of sinusoidal endothelial cells and sloughing of endothelial

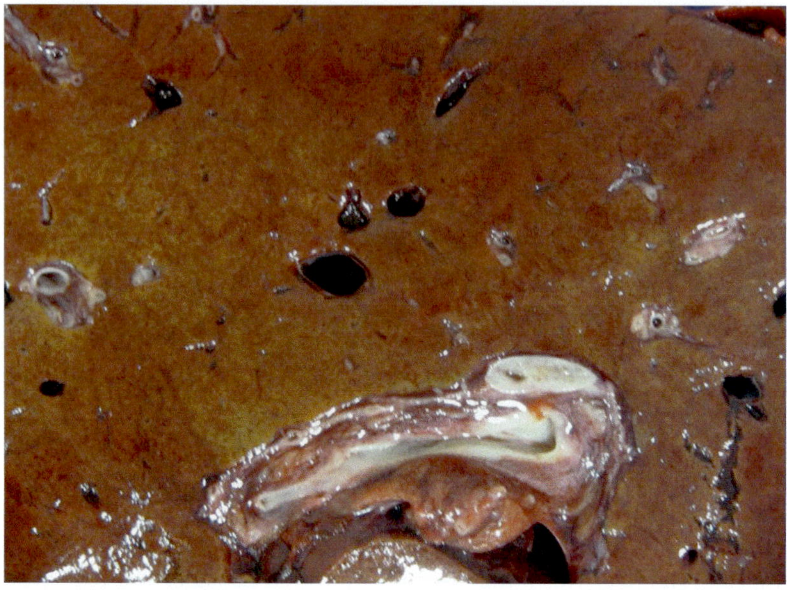

FIG. 5.15   This liver failed during transplant surgery. Centrilobular congestion and necrosis are grossly evident (same case as Fig. 5.14).

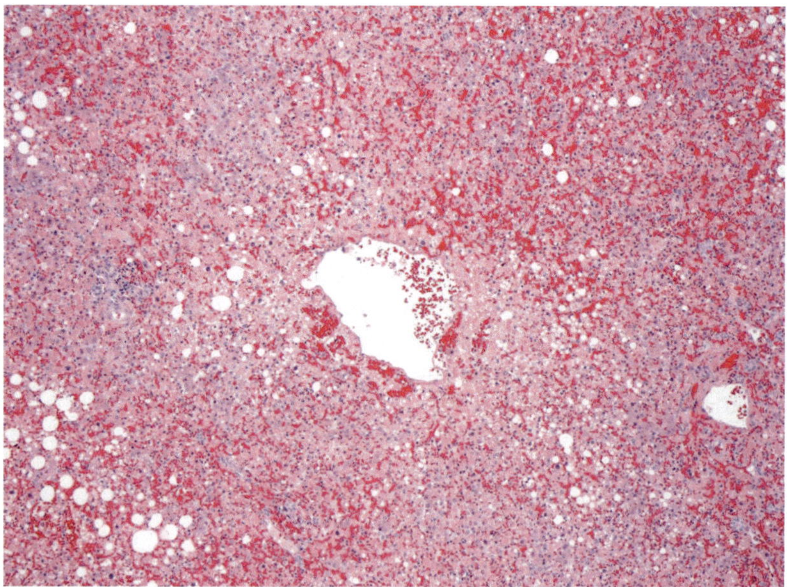

FIG. 5.16   The failed graft shows massive parenchymal necrosis (same case as Fig. 5.14).

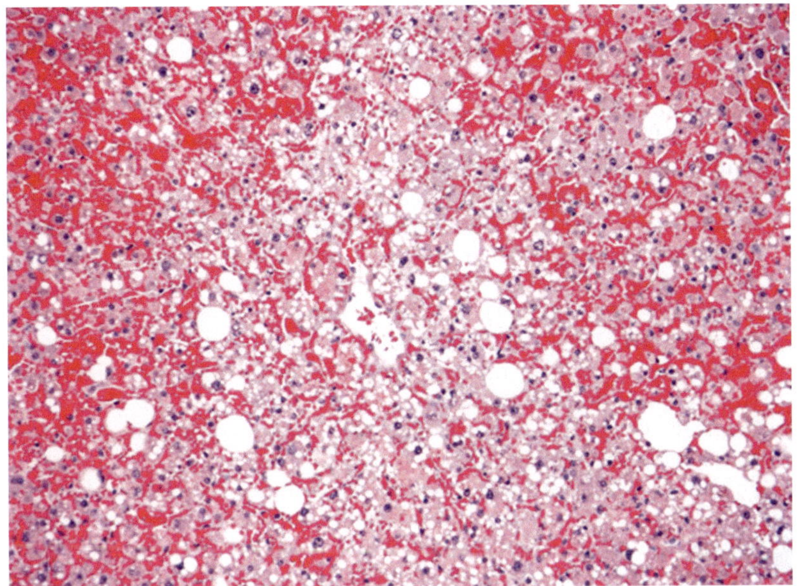

FIG. 5.17 The failed graft is largely necrotic with hemorrhage and steatosis, both of which are more prominent in a centrilobular distribution. Note a paucity of inflammation (same case as Fig. 5.14).

cells into vascular lumina [28]. Primary graft nonfunction is also a potential complication of severe macrovesicular steatosis, which impedes graft reperfusion and promotes ischemia. Ischemia-related hepatocyte death results in accumulation of large extracellular fat deposits that cause mechanical compression of the sinusoids and facilitate additional hepatocellular necrosis [28]. Hyperacute allograft rejection occurs in recipients who harbor preformed antidonor antibodies. It may occur immediately after transplantation or manifest several days after surgery. Some cases are heralded by a rapid rise in serum aminotransferase levels and serologic evidence of coagulopathy within 2 h of transplantation [26]. This type of rejection does not respond to immunosuppressive therapy and requires urgent retransplantation [28]. Hyperacute rejection results in fibrin deposition in hepatic sinusoids, which is evident within 2–6 h of transplantation. Diffuse neutrophilic infiltration and widespread congestion with massive necrosis ensue within 1 or 2 days. Well-developed hyperacute rejection closely resembles reperfusion injury and steatosis-related injury, so the diagnosis often relies on a combination of microscopic findings and clinical evidence. Demonstration of a presensitized state in the recipient and exclusion of other potential causes facilitate the diagnosis [28].

References

1. Busuttil RW, Tanaka K. The utility of marginal donors in liver transplantation. Liver Transpl. 2003;9(7):651–63.
2. Kauffman HM, McBride MA, Cherikh WS, Spain PC, Marks WH, Roza AM. Transplant tumor registry: donor related malignancies. Transplantation. 2002;74:358–62.
3. Morath C, Schwenger V, Schmidt J, Zeier M. Transmission of malignancy with solid organ transplants. Transplantation. 2005;80:S164–6.
4. Loren AW, Desai S, Gorman RC, Schuchter LM. Retransplantation of a cardiac allograft inadvertantly harvested from a donor with malignant melanoma. Transplantation. 2003;76:741–3.
5. Stephens JK, Everson GT, Elliot CL, et al. Fatal transfer of malignant melanoma from multiorgan donor to four allograft recipients. Transplantation. 2000;70:232–6.
6. Buell JF, Gross TG, Woodle ES. Malignancy after transplantation. Transplantation. 2005;80:S254.
7. Lipshutz GS, Baxter-Lowe LA, Nguyen T, Jones KD, Ascher NL, Feng S. Death from donor-transmitted malignancy despite emergency liver retransplantation. Liver Transpl. 2003;9:1102–7.
8. Takeda Y, Arii S, Kaido T, Niwano M, Moriga T, Mori A. Morphologic alteration of hepatocytes and sinuisoidal endothelial cells in rat fatty liver during cold preservation and the protective effect of hepatocyte growth factor. Transplantation. 1999;67:820–8.
9. Fukumori T, Ohkohchi N, Tsukamoto S, Satomi S. Why is fatty liver unsuitable for transplantation? Deterioration of mitochondrial ATP synthesis and sinusoidal structure during cold preservation of a liver with steatosis. Transpl Proc. 1997;29:412–5.
10. Fishbein TM, Fiel MI, Emre S, et al. Use of livers with microvesicular fat safely expands the donor pool. Transplantation. 1997;64(2):248–51.
11. Urena MAG, Ruiz-Delgado FC, Gonzalez EM, et al. Assessing risk of the use of livers with macro and microsteatosis in a liver transplant program. Transplant Proc. 1998;30:3288–91.
12. Adani GL, Baccarani U, Sainz-Barriga M, et al. The role of hepatic biopsy to detect macrovacuolar steatosis during liver procurement. Transplant Proc. 2006;38(5):1404–6.
13. Loinaz C, Gonzalez EM. Marginal donors in liver transplantation. Hepatogastroenterology. 2000;47(31):256–63.
14. Markin RS, Wisecarver JL, Radio SJ, et al. Frozen section evaluation of donor livers before transplantation. Transplantation. 1993;56(6):1403–9.
15. D'Alessandro E, Calabrese F, Gringeri E, Valente M. Frozen-section diagnosis in donor livers: error rate estimation of steatosis degree. Transplant Proc. 2010;42:2226–8.
16. Cieslak B, Lewandowski Z, Urban M, Ziarkiewicz-Wroblewska B, Krawczyk M. Microvesicular liver graft steatosis as a risk factor for initial poor function in relation to suboptimal donor parameters. Transpl Proc. 2009;41(8):2985–8.
17. Briceno J, Marchal T, Padillo J, Solorzano G, Pera C. Influence of marginal donors on liver preservation injury. Transplantation. 2002;74:522–6.

18. Reich DJ, Hong JC. Current status of donation after cardiac death liver transplantation. Curr Opin Organ Transplant. 2010;15(3):316–21.
19. Kakizoe S, Yanaga K, Starzl TE, Demetris AJ. Frozen section of liver biopsy for evaluation of liver allografts. Transplant Proc. 1990;22(2): 416–7.
20. Kakizoe S, Yanaga K, Starzl TE, Demetris AJ. Evaluation of protocol before transplanation and after reperfusion biopsies from human orthotopic liver allografts: considerations of preservation and early immunologic injury. Hepatology. 1990;11(6):932–41.
21. Zamboni F, Franchello A, David E, et al. Effect of macro-vesicular steatosis and other donor and recipient characteristics on the outcome of liver transplantation. Clin Transplant. 2001;15:53–7.
22. Velidedeoglu E, Desai NM, Campos L, et al. The outcome of liver grafts procured from hepatitis C-positive donors. Transplantation. 2002;73(4):582–7.
23. Demetris AJ, Crawford JM, Minervini MI, et al. Transplantation pathology of the liver. In: Odze RD, Goldblum JR, editors. Surgical pathology of the GI tract, liver, biliary tract, and pancreas. Philadelphia: Saunders Elsevier; 2009. p. 1169–229.
24. Jeon H, Lee S-G. Living donor liver transplantation. Curr Opin Organ Transplant. 2010;15:283–7.
25. Gruttadauria S, di Francesco F, Vizzini GB, et al. Early graft dysfunction following adult-to-adult living-related liver transplantation: predictive factors and outcomes. World J Gastroenterol. 2009;15(36):4556–60.
26. Bennett-Guerrero E, Feierman DE, Barclay GR, et al. Preoperative and intraoperative predictors of postoperative morbidity, poor graft function, and early rejection in 190 patients undergoing liver transplantation. Arch Surg. 2001;136:1177–83.
27. Bzeizi KI, Jalan R, Plevris JN, Hayes PC. Primary graft dysfunction after liver transplantation: from pathogenesis to prevention. Liver Transpl Surg. 1997;3(2):137–48.
28. Hubscher SG, Portmann BC. Transplantation pathology. In: MacSween RNM, Burt AD, Portmann BC, Ishak KG, Scheuer PJ, Anthony PP, editors. Pathology of the liver. 4th ed. London: Churchill Livingstone; 2002. p. 885–941.
29. Scheuer PJ. Classification of chronic viral hepatitis: a need for reassessment. J Hepatol. 1991;13:372–4.

Chapter 6
Intraoperative Evaluation of the Extrahepatic Biliary Tree and Ampulla of Vater

INTRODUCTION

Carcinomas of the extrahepatic biliary tree and ampulla of Vater are usually diagnosed preoperatively *via* cytologic brushing or biopsy, so frozen sections of these tumors are limited to evaluation of bile duct margins. These specimens may require orientation by the surgeon in order to identify the appropriate margins for assessment. Tumors of the proximal extrahepatic biliary tree require resection of bile ducts and possibly part of the liver, whereas those of the distal common bile duct and ampulla are resected *via* pancreaticoduodenectomy. Benign inflammatory conditions of bile ducts can cause strictures that simulate the radiographic appearance of malignancy. These disorders induce reactive epithelial cell changes that may not be definitively classified by cytologic evaluation or preoperative biopsy. Thus, they are intraoperatively sampled and submitted for frozen section analysis. The purpose of this chapter is to discuss the histologic features of benign inflammatory disorders of the extrahepatic bile ducts, neoplasms of the bile ducts and ampulla of Vater, and issues related to evaluation of margins on cancer resection specimens.

NONNEOPLASTIC MIMICS OF EXTRAHEPATIC CHOLANGIOCARCINOMA

Benign etiologies account for 5–10% of surgically treated extrahepatic biliary strictures and the remainder represent invasive adenocarcinomas [1–5]. Benign and malignant biliary strictures cause similar signs and symptoms related to biliary obstruction.

113

R.K. Yantiss (ed.), *Frozen Section Library: Liver, Extrahepatic Biliary Tree and Gallbladder*, Frozen Section Library, DOI 10.1007/978-1-4614-0043-1_6,
© Springer Science+Business Media, LLC 2011

They are radiographically indistinguishable in many cases and both display increased metabolic activity on positron emission tomography [6]. Biopsies of benign bile duct strictures usually show inflammation and fibrosis, although some disorders produce characteristic microscopic changes that lead to a specific diagnosis in the appropriate clinical context. Frozen sections obtained from benign bile ducts may be difficult to evaluate because the normal lobular architecture of epithelial elements may be somewhat distorted by inflammation, ulcers, and fibrosis (Fig. 6.1). These changes are more severe in bile duct strictures that show a greater degree of gland distortion, mural inflammation, and scar (Fig. 6.2). However, the mural epithelial elements display only minimal cytologic atypia and are invested in a cuff of slightly cellular stroma (Fig. 6.3). Placement of biliary stents and choledocholithiasis causes mucosal erosions and regenerative changes in adjacent intact epithelium, including mucin depletion and nuclear prominence (Fig. 6.4).

Isolated Benign Strictures

Isolated benign strictures of the extrahepatic ducts develop following biliary surgery, cholecystectomy, or recurrent episodes

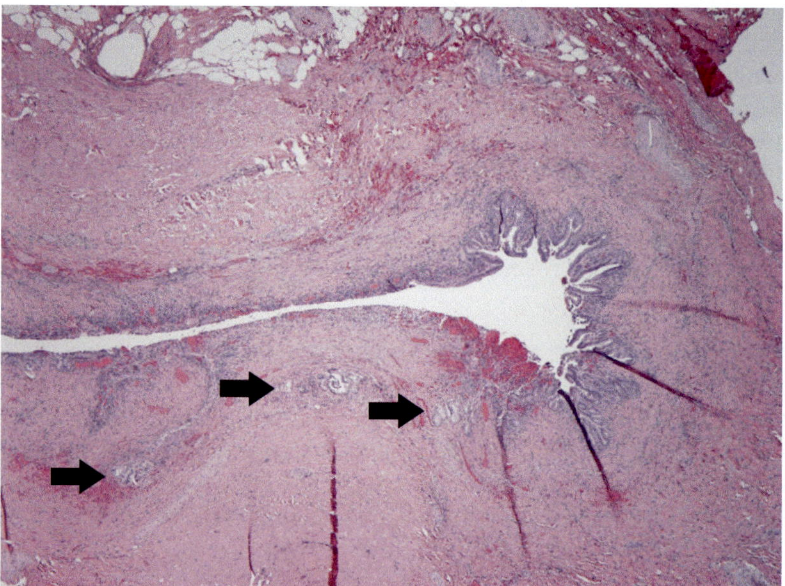

FIG. 6.1 Benign bile ducts are lined by a single layer of epithelium and have occasional lobules of periductal glands in the wall (*arrows*).

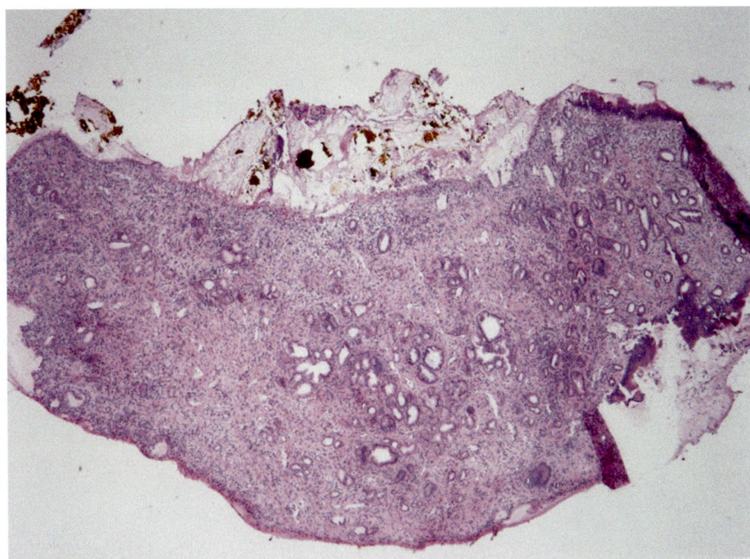

FIG. 6.2 A benign bile duct stricture shows mural fibrosis with inflammation that expands and distorts the architecture of periductal glands. However, the glands maintain a vaguely lobular arrangement and are not associated with desmoplasia.

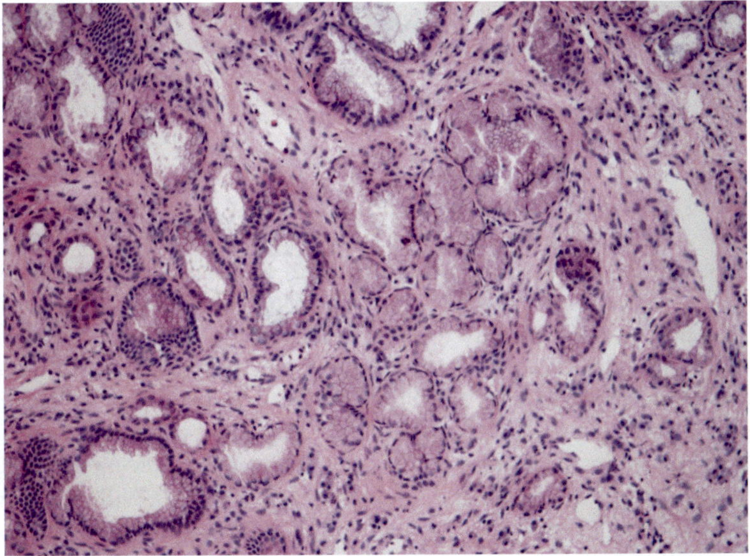

FIG. 6.3 Benign periductal glands contain cuboidal epithelial cells with round, basally located nuclei and abundant mucinous cytoplasm. They are arranged in lobules surrounded by a cuff of cellular stroma (same case as Fig. 6.2).

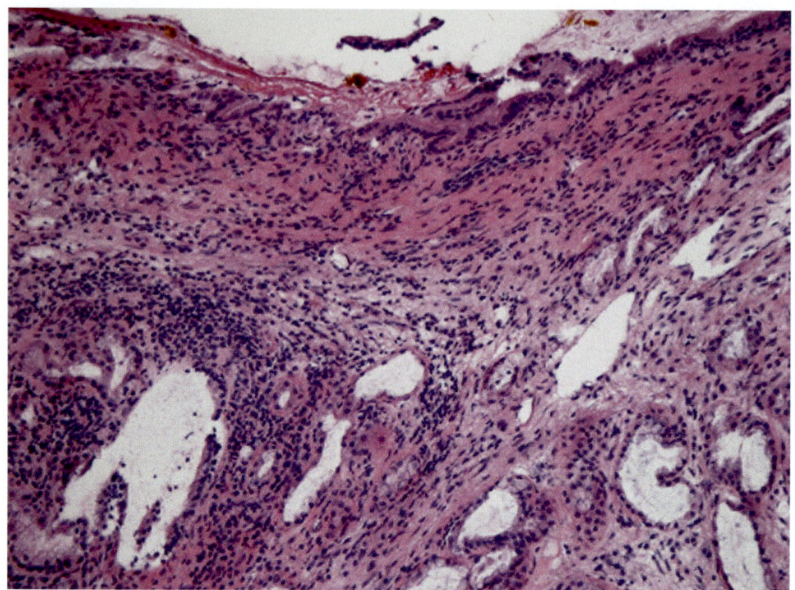

FIG. 6.4 The luminal epithelium of the scarred duct is partially denuded and the remaining epithelial cells show mucin depletion. Their nuclei are slightly enlarged, but basally located (same case as Figs. 6.2 and 6.3).

of cholangitis [7, 8]. Stenotic segments contain paucicellular scar tissue in the wall with variable numbers of inflammatory cells (Fig. 6.5). Proliferating glands are arranged in lobules and contain polarized cuboidal cells with neutral mucin and minimal, if any, cytologic atypia (Figs. 6.6 and 6.7).

Primary Sclerosing Cholangitis

Primary sclerosing cholangitis is a chronic stricturing disease of the intra- and extrahepatic bile ducts that is diagnosed radiographically. It produces a characteristic "beaded" appearance on endoscopic retrograde cholangiopancreatography due to progressive scarring of extrahepatic bile ducts and destruction of intrahepatic ducts (Fig. 6.8) [9]. Approximately 80% of patients have underlying inflammatory bowel disease (IBD) and first-degree relatives of IBD patients are at increased risk for developing this disease [10]. Most patients with primary sclerosing cholangitis will either die of disease or require liver transplantation within 12–18 years of presentation [11]. They are also at increased risk (4–14%) for cholangiocarcinoma of the intra- or extrahepatic bile ducts [12]. Unfortunately, the radiographic surveillance of patients with primary sclerosing cholangitis for malignant strictures is challenging

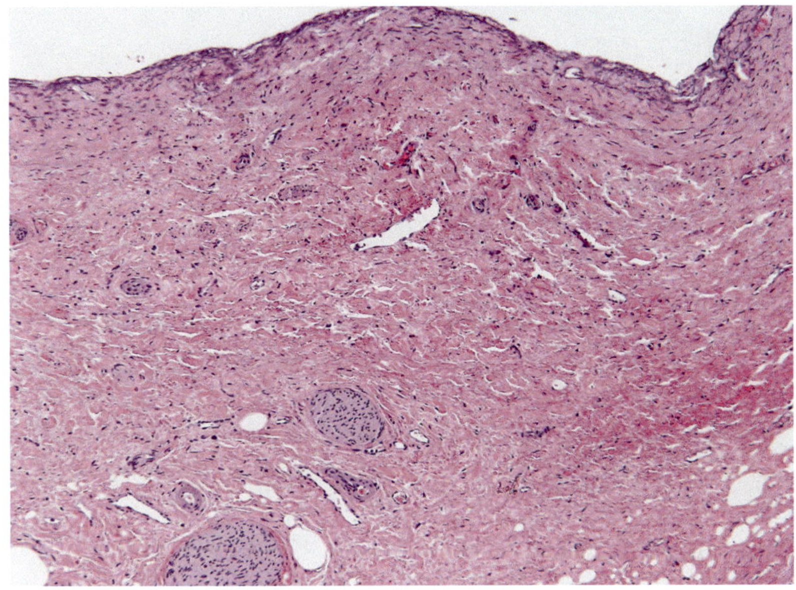

FIG. 6.5 Isolated benign bile duct strictures show dense mural fibrosis. Collagen bundles interrupt the muscularis and a superficial sparse inflammatory infiltrate is present.

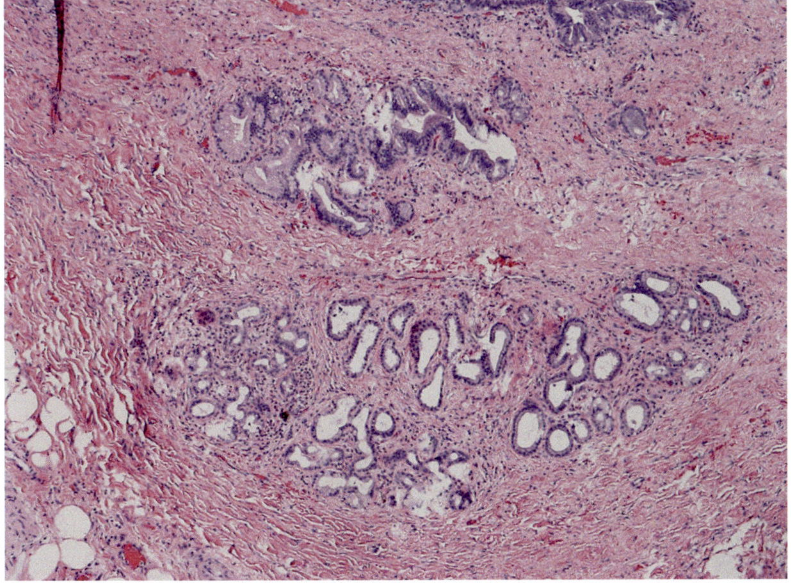

FIG. 6.6 Benign periductal glands in the bile duct walls maintain their lobular architecture despite the presence of fibrosis and inflammation.

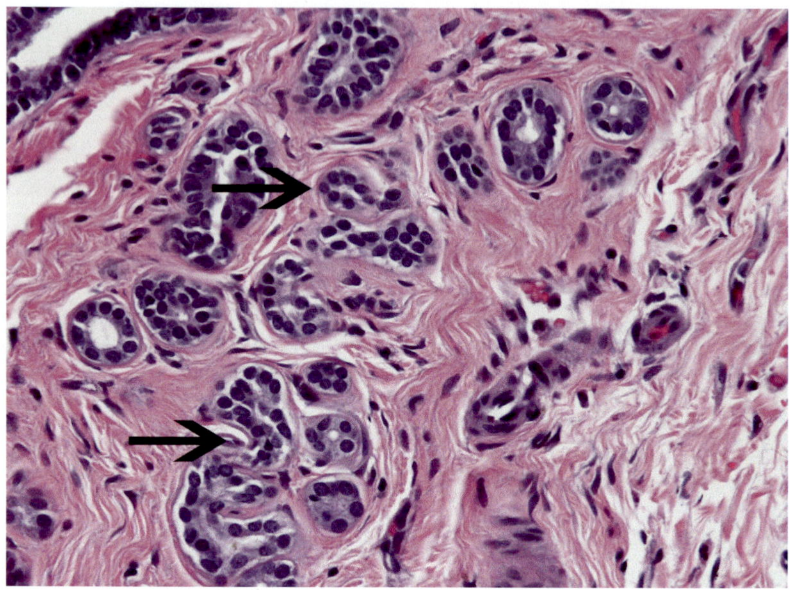

FIG. 6.7 Lobules of periductal glands are distorted and compressed by mural fibrosis. These angulated glands (*arrows*) may be worrisome for malignancy, but they contain cells with basal nuclei and lack cytologic atypia.

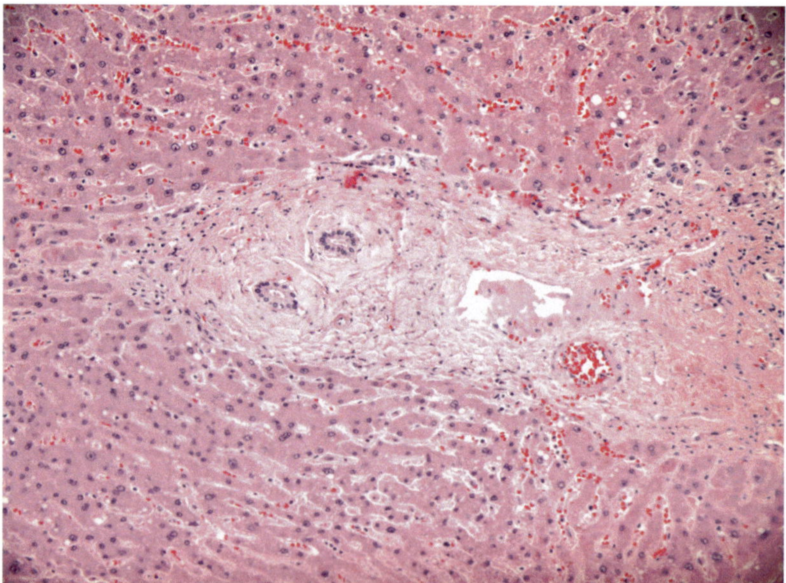

FIG. 6.8 Primary sclerosing cholangitis results in progressive concentric fibrosis surrounding bile ducts in the liver and extrahepatic biliary tree.

because many carcinomas are radiographically indistinguishable from benign strictures. Primary sclerosing cholangitis does not cause specific histologic changes in extrahepatic bile duct strictures, which appear as mural scars with variable numbers of lymphocytes and plasma cells in the wall and mucosa. Ulcers, erosions, and neutrophils may also be present, in which case the surface epithelial cells show regenerative, or reactive, atypia.

Lymphoplasmacytic Sclerosing Cholangitis

Lymphoplasmacytic sclerosing cholangitis is one member of a family of systemic diseases characterized by elevated serum IgG4 levels and increased numbers of IgG4-positive plasma cells. Pertinent laboratory findings include elevated alkaline phosphatase, and transaminase levels, as well as high titers of immunoglobulins and circulating autoantibodies. IgG4-related disorders respond well to corticosteroid therapy, suggesting that they are immune-mediated [13, 14]. These diseases occur in the pancreas, bile ducts, gallbladder, gastrointestinal tract, salivary glands, bone marrow, and other sites [15]. Approximately 60–80% of patients with pancreatic disease (autoimmune pancreatitis) also have involvement of the distal bile duct [16].

Lymphoplasmacytic sclerosing cholangitis may not be suspected until frozen section evaluation because its clinical features closely parallel to those of malignant biliary strictures and preoperative evaluation is rarely conclusive. Resected specimens contain segmental bile duct strictures with prestenotic duct dilatation. Histologic sections reveal dense fibrosis associated with subepithelial plasma cell-rich inflammatory cell infiltrates (Fig. 6.9). Lymphocytes are present in the duct epithelium, which may display mild cytologic atypia (Figs. 6.10 and 6.11). Obliterative phlebitis in the bile duct wall is characteristic, but not uniformly present. Immunohistochemical stains for IgG4-positive plasma cells usually demonstrate an average of 10 IgG4-positive cells per high-power field [17].

CHOLEDOCHAL CYSTS

Choledochal cysts are congenital cystic dilatations of the bile ducts. They are relatively rare in western countries compared to Asian populations. Most extrahepatic cysts occur proximal to an abnormal confluence of the common bile duct and main pancreatic duct. Choledochal cysts are usually diagnosed in children, but approximately 20% cause symptoms in adulthood. Clinical symptoms are related to cholangitis or pancreatitis that may prompt surgery, at which time a frozen section evaluation could be requested [18]. Choledochal cysts are classified based on their number and anatomic location. Type I cysts account for 95% of cases and are

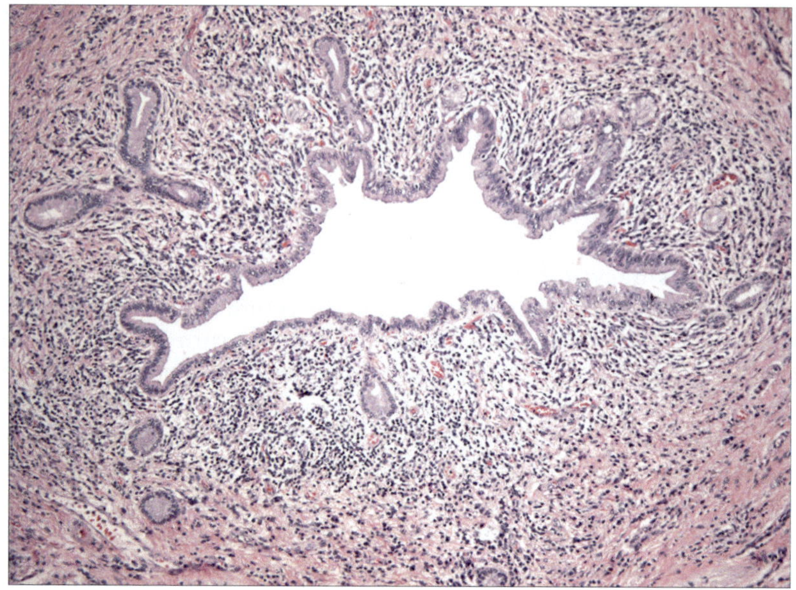

FIG. 6.9 A dense, plasma cell-rich inflammatory infiltrate surrounds a duct in a patient with lymphoplasmacytic sclerosing cholangitis and pancreatitis.

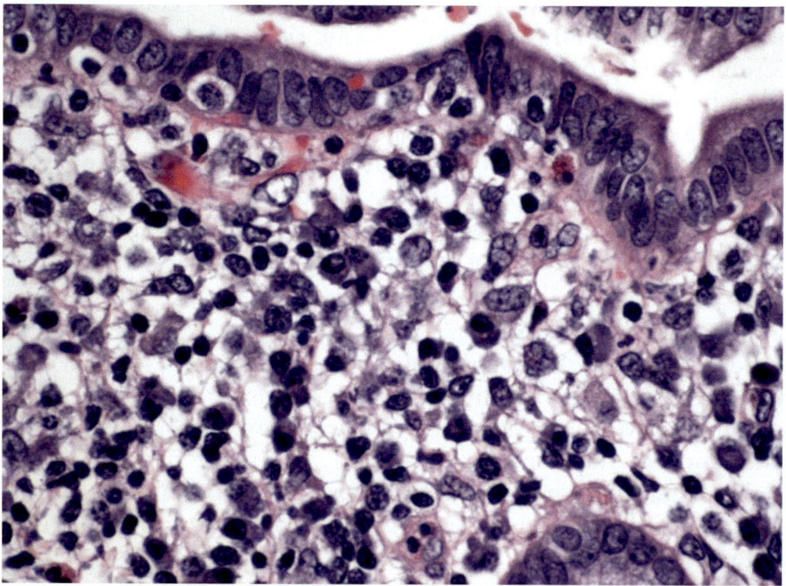

FIG. 6.10 Numerous lymphocytes and plasma cells are present in the biliary mucosa. Intraepithelial lymphocytes are also apparent (same case as Fig. 6.9).

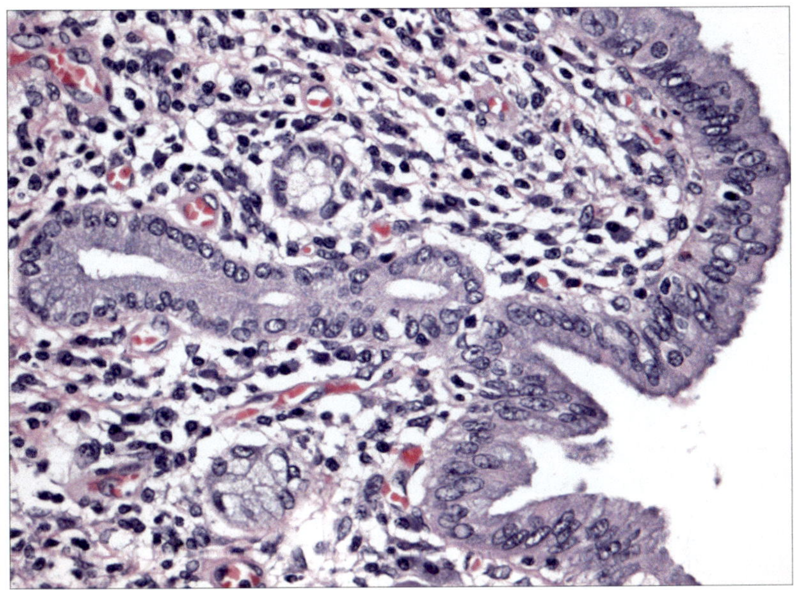

Fɪɢ. 6.11 Inflammation-induced nuclear enlargement and pseudostratification in biliary epithelial cells mimics dysplasia (same case as Figs. 6.9 and 6.10).

fusiform dilatations of the common hepatic duct or common bile duct. Type II cysts are true diverticula of the extrahepatic bile ducts. Type III cysts are confined to the duodenal wall (choledochocele) and type IV cysts are multifocal within the liver and/or extrahepatic biliary tree. Type V choledochal cysts (Caroli's disease) are multifocal intrahepatic lesions (Fig. 6.12) [19]. Surgery usually involves resection of the affected bile ducts with subsequent anastomosis of the biliary tree to the jejunum, although patients with Caroli's disease require partial hepatic resection or liver transplantation [18]. Choledochal cysts have a firm, fibrotic wall and contain variable quantities of bile. The cysts are lined by biliary-type epithelium, although the surface may be denuded in older patients. The wall contains disorganized smooth muscle bundles with fibrous tissue and dystrophic calcifications in some cases (Figs. 6.13 and 6.14). Choledochal cysts are subject to chronic bile stasis and infection, so they are at risk for inflammation-induced neoplasia. The risk of invasive adenocarcinoma is reported to be approximately 30% in adults [20]. Frozen section analysis may be requested when surgeons encounter abnormally thickened, polypoid, or discolored areas in choledochal cysts [20, 21].

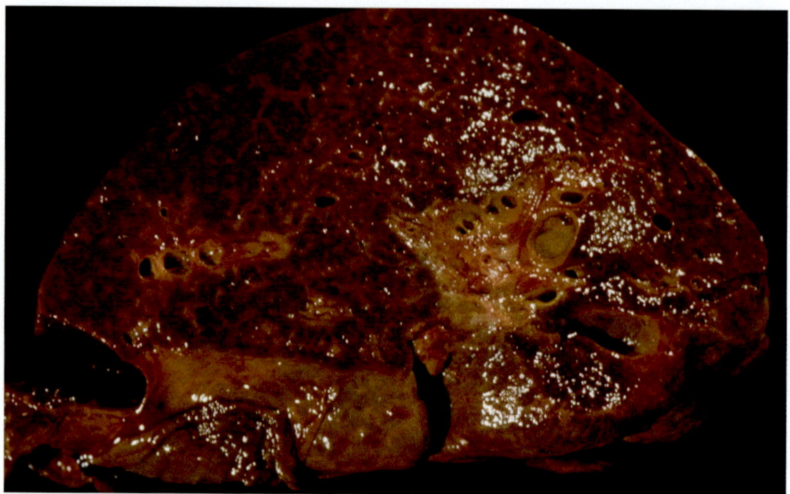

FIG. 6.12 Multiple intrahepatic bile ducts are cystically dilated in this patient with Caroli's disease.

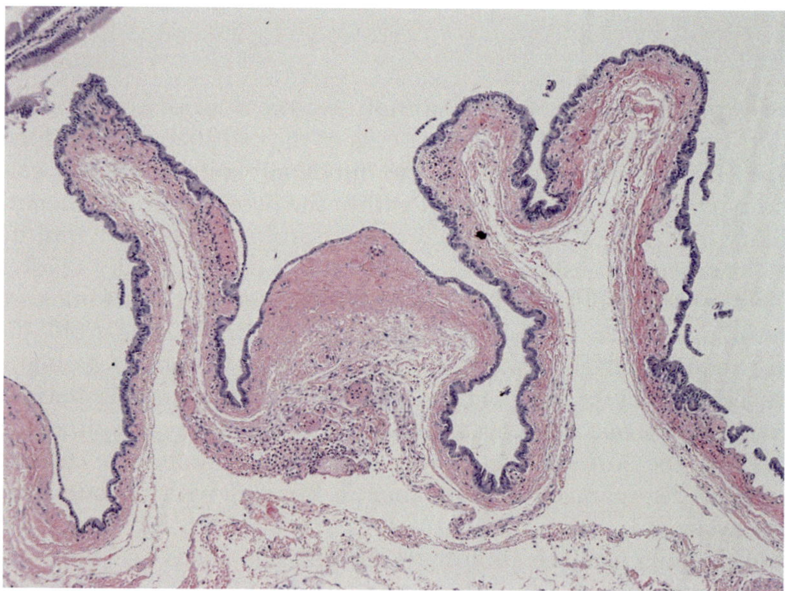

FIG. 6.13 The wall of a choledochal cyst consists of smooth muscle bundles and fibrous tissue. A single layer of biliary epithelium lines the lumen.

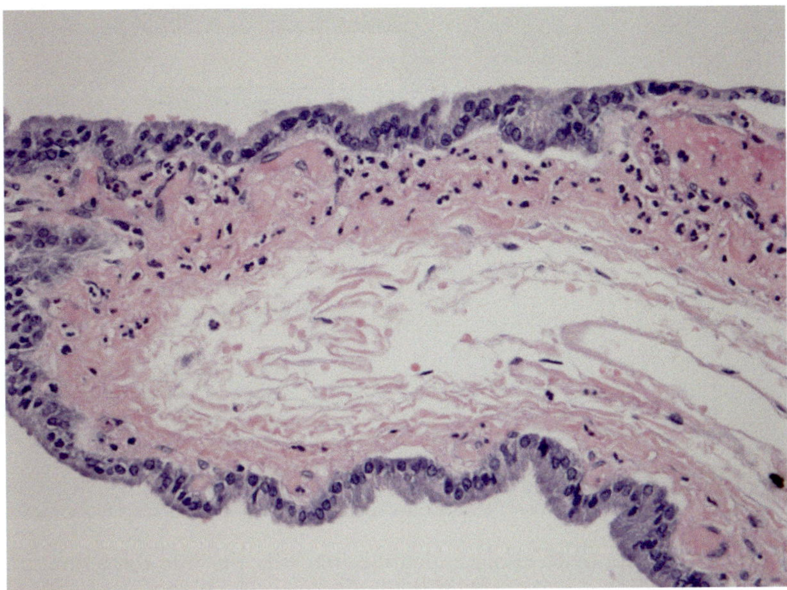

FIG. 6.14 The epithelium of this choledochal cyst is arranged in a single layer. The cells are cuboidal-to-columnar in shape and show slight nuclear enlargement owing to acute inflammation (same case as Fig. 6.13).

EXTRAHEPATIC CHOLANGIOCARCINOMA

Risk factors for extrahepatic bile duct carcinomas include primary sclerosing cholangitis, ulcerative colitis, an abnormal choledocho-pancreatic junction, choledochal cysts (including Caroli's disease), and infestation with liver flukes [22]. Extrahepatic cholangiocarcinomas are aggressive tumors with a poor prognosis. The 5-year survival rate is only 20–40% following attempted curative resection [23]. For staging purposes, carcinomas are divided into three groups based on their anatomic location. Tumors above the cystic duct junction and those involving the right or left hepatic ducts, the common hepatic duct, or the cystic duct are proximal cholangiocarcinomas. Tumors that occur distal to the cystic duct junction and involve the middle third of the extrahepatic biliary tree are mid-duct carcinomas and those that affect the distal half of the common bile duct are classified as distal cholangiocarcinomas [24].

Carcinomas of the extrahepatic bile ducts are diffusely infiltrative and cause strictures with, or without, a polypoid luminal component (Fig. 6.15). Most are of pancreatobiliary type and contain malignant glands associated with desmoplastic stroma,

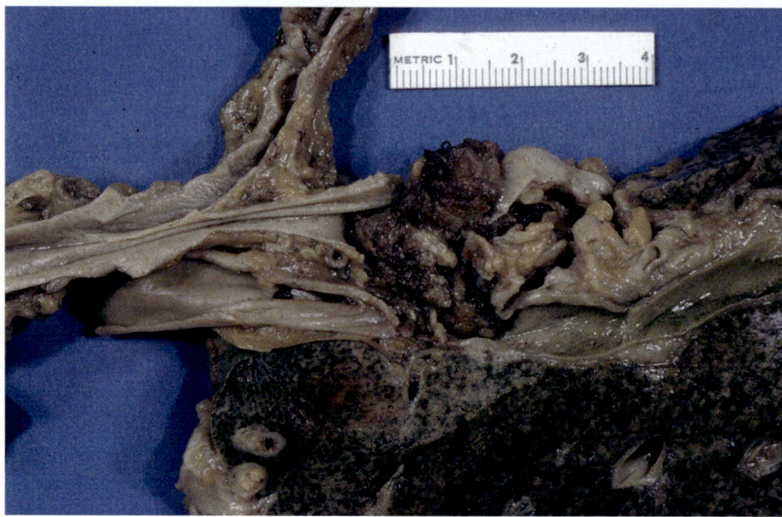

FIG. 6.15 An exophytic cholangiocarcinoma fills the bile duct lumen at the confluence of the right and left hepatic ducts. The hepatic parenchyma is bile stained due to obstruction (photograph courtesy of Dr. Carrie Besanceney).

although some tumors are polypoid with a complex papillary architecture (Fig. 6.16) [22, 25].

Margin Assessment and Specimen Preparation

Resection specimens for proximal and mid-duct cancers include a portion of the biliary tree, the gallbladder, and attached soft tissue with lymph nodes. Orientation should be confirmed by the surgeon prior to sectioning, in order to ensure that the margins are appropriately designated. Resection specimens are opened longitudinally along the duct to evaluate tumor extent. Histologic samples include cross sections of the duct to evaluate depth of invasion and all lymph nodes present in periductal fat. Resections for proximal tumors may include a portion of liver, so the hepatic parenchymal margin should be representatively submitted. Carcinomas of the distal common bile duct are resected *via* pancreaticoduodenectomy. These specimens include a segment of duodenum with or without a portion of stomach, the proximal pancreas, and distal extrapancreatic bile duct. The duodenum is opened opposite the ampulla, which is subsequently probed and opened along the bile duct. Photographs document the relationship between the tumor, pancreas, ampulla, and common bile duct.

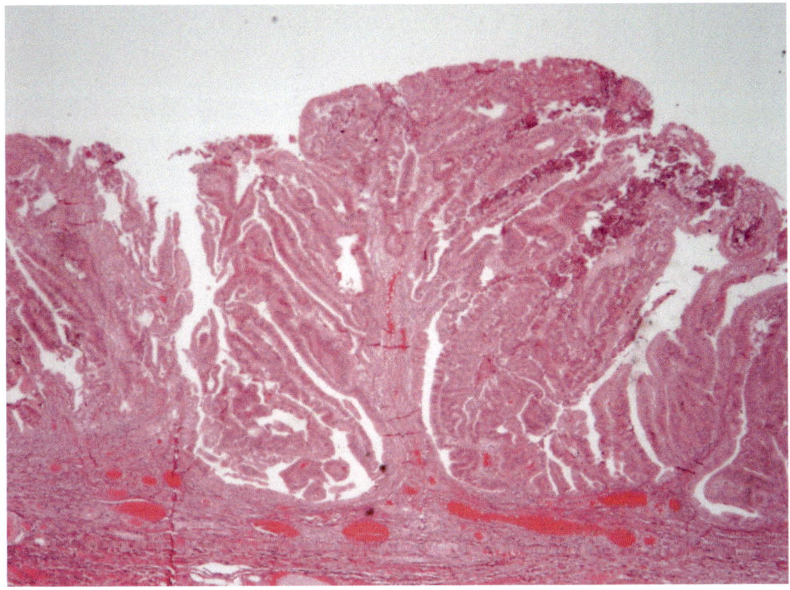

FIG. 6.16 This extrahepatic cholangiocarcinoma displays complex papillary architecture and the tumor protrudes into the lumen.

Bile duct margins are usually shaved and examined *en face*, but tumors within 0.2 cm of the margin may be sectioned perpendicularly to assess clearance. Poor prognosis and high rates of anastomotic recurrence have been observed in patients with positive bile duct margins, so intraoperative recognition of carcinoma at the resection margin is important [26]. Features that aid the evaluation of bile duct margins are enumerated in Table 6.1. Benign bile ducts contain a single layer of cuboidal-to-columnar epithelial cells at the mucosal surface and lobules of glands in the wall (Figs. 6.17 and 6.18). The glands are lined by cells with abundant cytoplasm, basal nuclei, and minimal atypia (Fig. 6.19). Inflammation-induced atypia, including slight nuclear enlargement, prominent nucleoli, and occasional mitoses, are seen in ulcers and in patients who have undergone prior manipulation of the bile duct. For this reason, one should always be cautious when making a diagnosis of malignancy or dysplasia in the setting of inflammation (Fig. 6.20). Most inflamed bile ducts show a spectrum of cytologic changes ranging from minimal to mild, or moderate, atypia, whereas neoplasia represents a second population of cells in an otherwise benign background. Carcinomas invade the bile duct mucosa or, more frequently, the wall. Mucosal neoplasia

TABLE 6.1 Distinguishing features of benign and malignant epithelium in bile duct margins.

Features	Benign glands	Adenocarcinoma
Mucosal changes		
Ulcer	May be present	Usually absent
Inflammation	May be present	Usually absent
Surface maturation of the epithelium	Present	Absent
Architecture of mucosal epithelium	Flat	Flat or complex
		Papillae
		Micropapillae
		Cribriform
Arrangement of glands	Lobules	Irregular distribution
Epithelial cell features		
Distribution of cytologic atypia	Spectrum of cytologic changes ranging from clearly benign to atypical	Two discrete populations of benign and atypical cells
Nuclear abnormalities	Mild to moderate	Moderate to severe
Nuclear variability	Absent or minimal	4:1 variation in nuclear size
Nucleoli	Inconspicuous	Variable, but may be large
Mitotic figures	Occasional	Numerous
Necrosis	Absent	May be present
Stroma	Fibrosis or smooth muscle	Desmoplasia

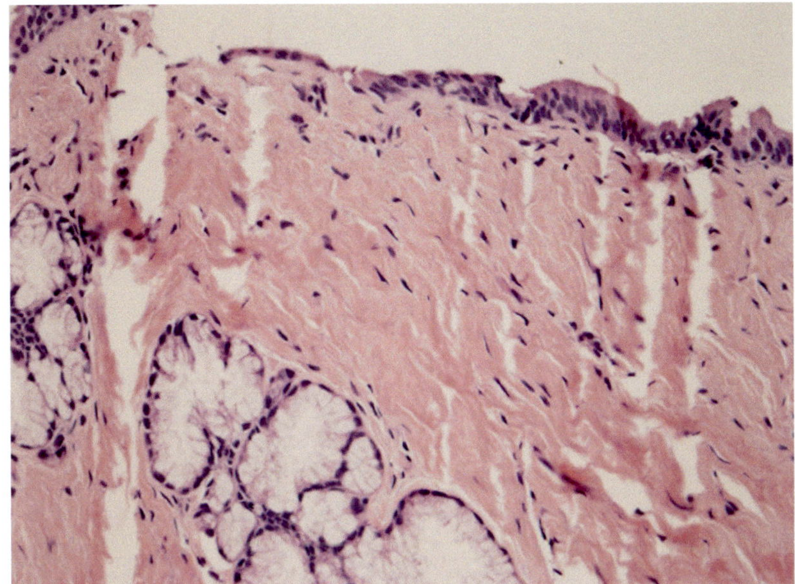

FIG. 6.17 Negative bile duct margins contain normal-appearing biliary epithelium in the mucosa and lobules of mucinous periductal glands.

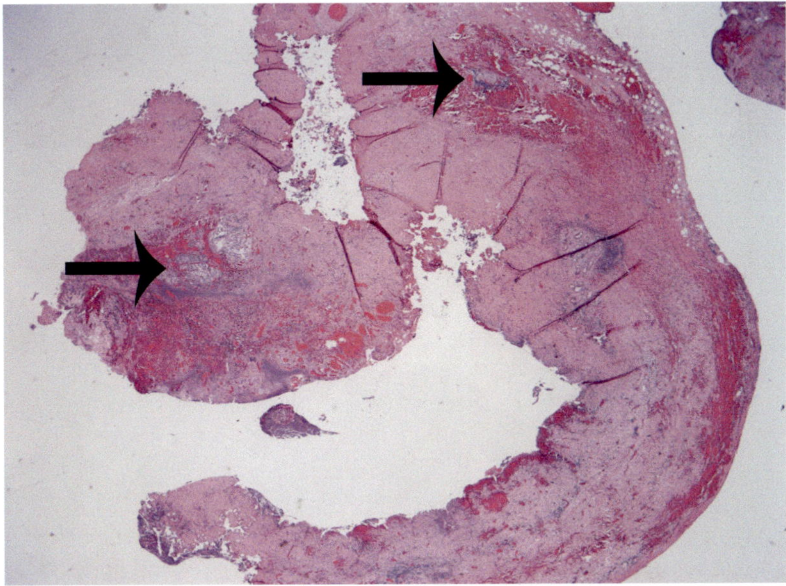

FIG. 6.18 The bile duct margin from a patient with carcinoma is negative for malignancy. It shows denuded mucosa and round aggregates of benign glands in the wall (*arrows*).

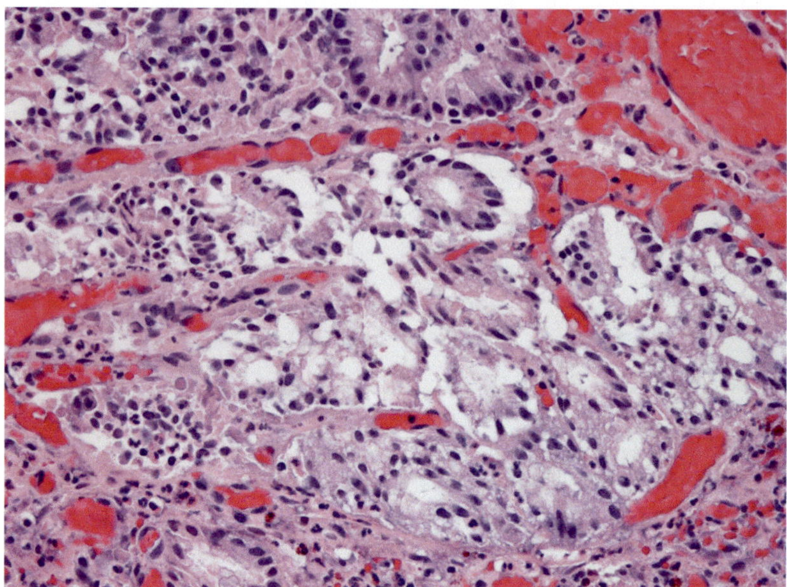

FIG. 6.19 Periductal glands are small and round with smooth, basally located nuclei and eosinophilic cytoplasm (same case as Fig. 6.18).

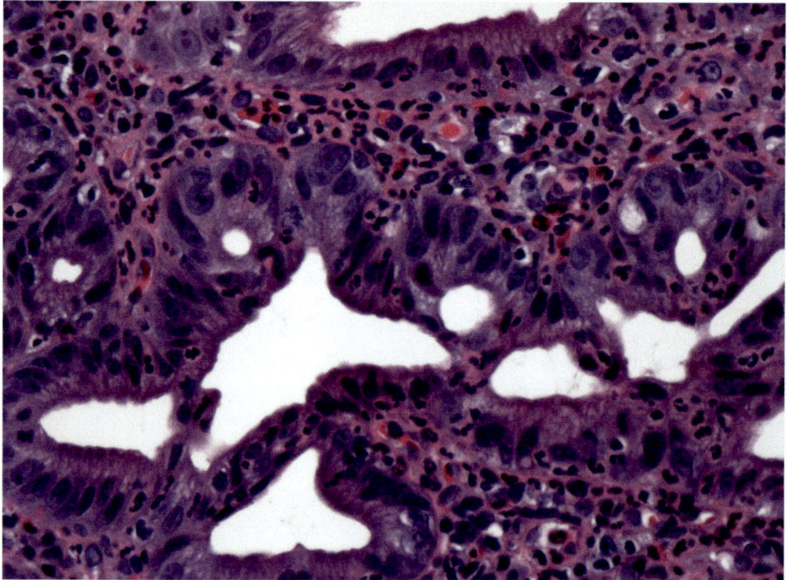

FIG. 6.20 Inflammation-induced biliary atypia may be both architectural and cytologic. These glands have a cribriform appearance and contain mucin-depleted cells with large nuclei and nucleoli. Intraepithelial neutrophils are present.

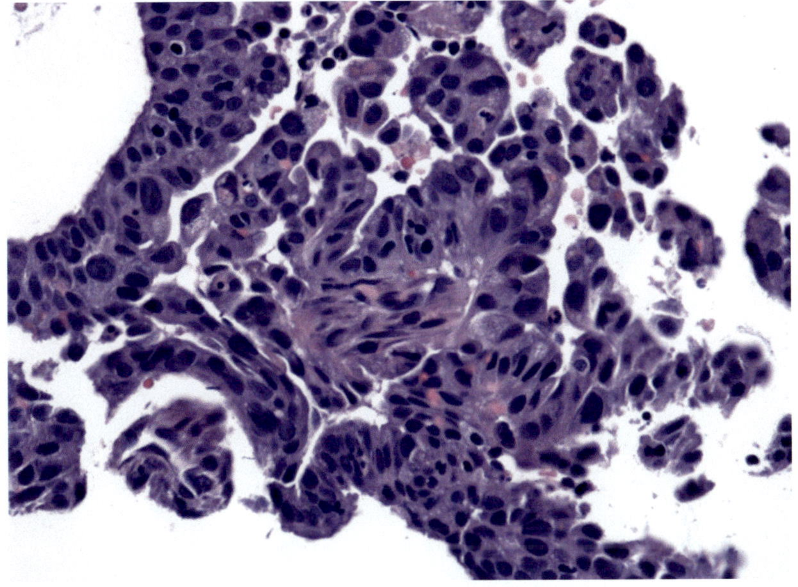

FIG. 6.21 Carcinoma in the bile duct shows a complex proliferation of high-grade cells.

in frozen sections of duct margins reflects either *de novo* dysplasia or colonization by carcinoma. It may be flat but is usually architecturally complex with micropapillae and buds of high-grade, dyshesive epithelial cells in the lumen (Figs. 6.21 and 6.22). Cholangiocarcinomas consist of angulated glands invested by desmoplastic stroma that diffusely infiltrate the bile duct wall. The tumor cells contain variable amounts of eosinophilic or basophilic cytoplasm with enlarged, stratified nuclei and numerous mitotic figures (Fig. 6.23). Perineural invasion is common and, when present, is a helpful clue to the diagnosis (Figs. 6.24 and 6.25).

FROZEN SECTION EVALUATION OF THE AMPULLA OF VATER

The ampulla of Vater is formed by the confluence of the common bile duct, pancreatic duct, and small intestine, creating complex microanatomy that juxtaposes glands, ductal epithelium, and muscularis mucosae. It is a common site for neoplasia relative to the rest of the small intestine [27]. Ampullary adenomas are morphologically similar to their colonic counterparts and display a tubular or villous architecture (Fig. 6.26). The criteria for grading dysplasia in ampullary adenomas are the same as those for the colon. Low-grade dysplasia is characterized by the presence of

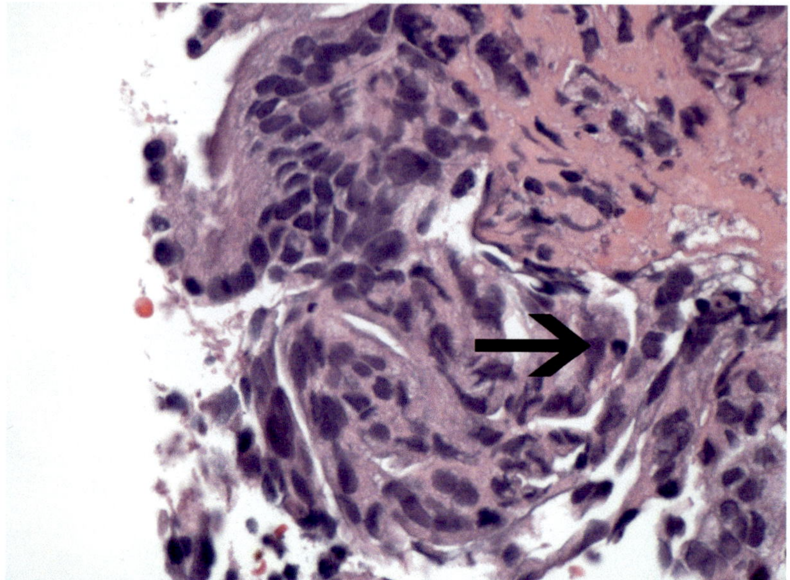

FIG. 6.22   Crushed carcinoma cells are crowded and show a high degree of nuclear variability with some mitotic figures (*arrow*).

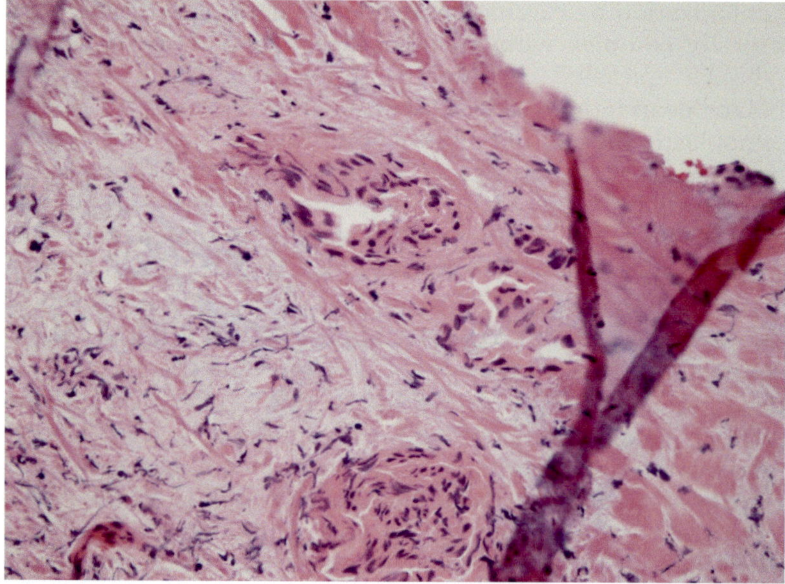

FIG. 6.23   The neoplastic glands are angulated and contain cells with nuclear hyperchromasia and pleomorphism.

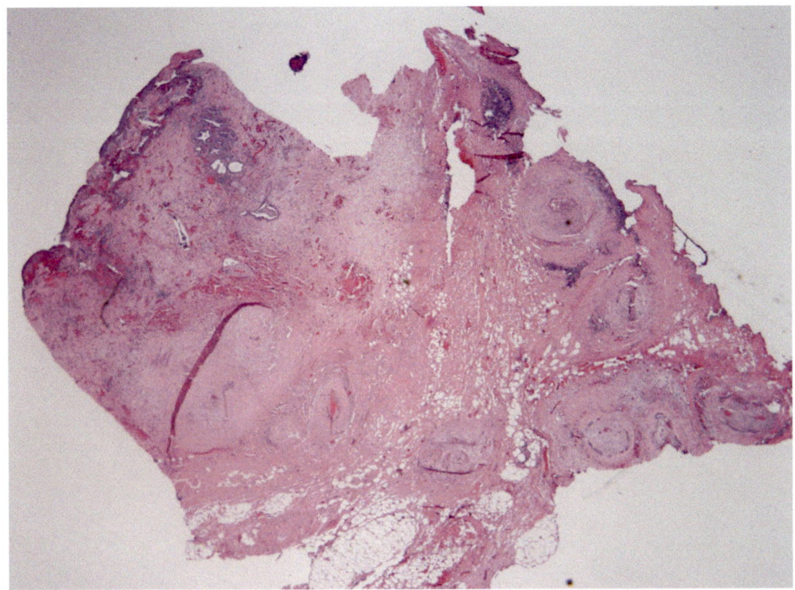

FIG. 6.24 Benign periductal glands are present adjacent to the mucosa (*left*). Malignant glands surround nerves (*right*) in the wall (same case Fig. 6.23).

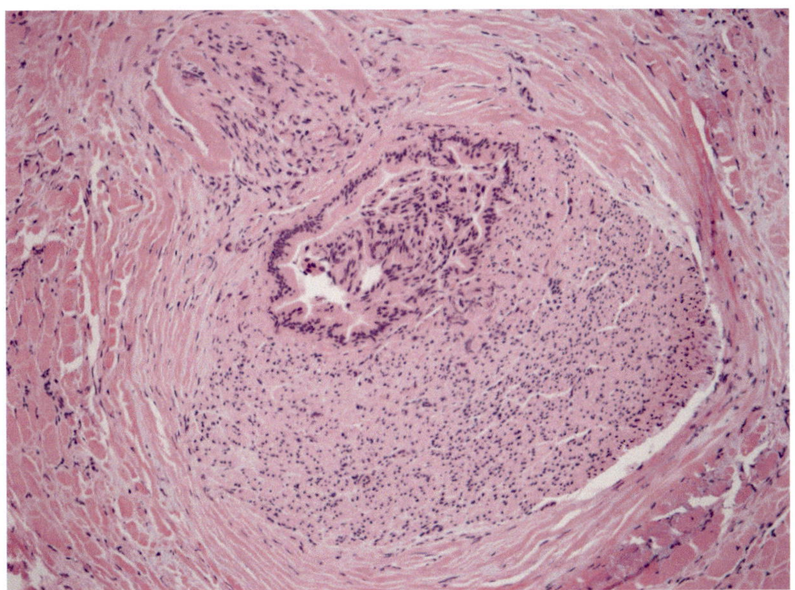

FIG. 6.25 Tumor cells are present in mural nerves (same case as Figs. 6.23 and 6.24).

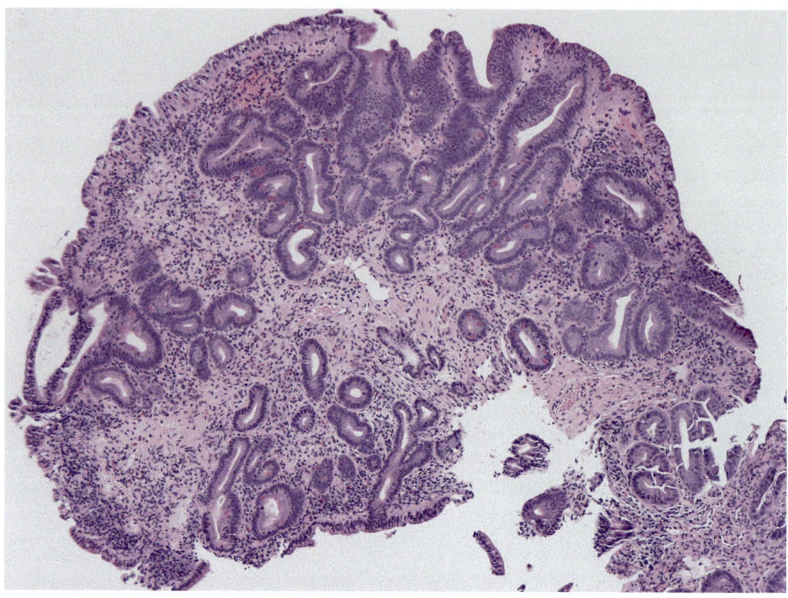

FIG. 6.26 This ampullary adenoma contains irregularly shaped and crowded glands.

nuclear hyperchromasia, elongation, and pseudostratification in the absence of architectural complexity (Fig. 6.27). High-grade dysplasia shows architectural and cytologic abnormalities. The neoplastic cells grow on delicate fibrovascular fronds or appear as micropapillae. Glands contain cribriform spaces and cells with nucleomegaly and prominent nucleoli. Mitotic figures and apoptotic debris are readily identified (Fig. 6.28). Most ampullary carcinomas are of intestinal type and display an expansile growth pattern of malignant glands that irregularly infiltrate the ampulla and elicit a desmoplastic reaction (Fig. 6.29) [28]. Approximately 30% are pancreatobiliary-type tumors that have a strictured gross appearance and contain small infiltrating ducts and single cells (Figs. 6.30 and 6.31). Most ampullary adenomas are amenable to endoscopic removal or ampullectomy, whereas invasive adenocarcinomas require pancreaticoduodenectomy. Thus, the clinician may request intraoperative consultation to exclude the possibility of invasive adenocarcinoma if a limited procedure is planned [29].

Evaluating frozen sections from tumors of the ampulla is challenging in some situations. Adenomas may colonize the deep ampullary glands, thereby simulating invasive carcinoma (Fig. 6.32). Clues that suggest a benign diagnosis include the lobular architecture of neoplastic elements and their cytologic similarity to cells in the overlying adenoma. The dysplastic glands are surrounded by a rim

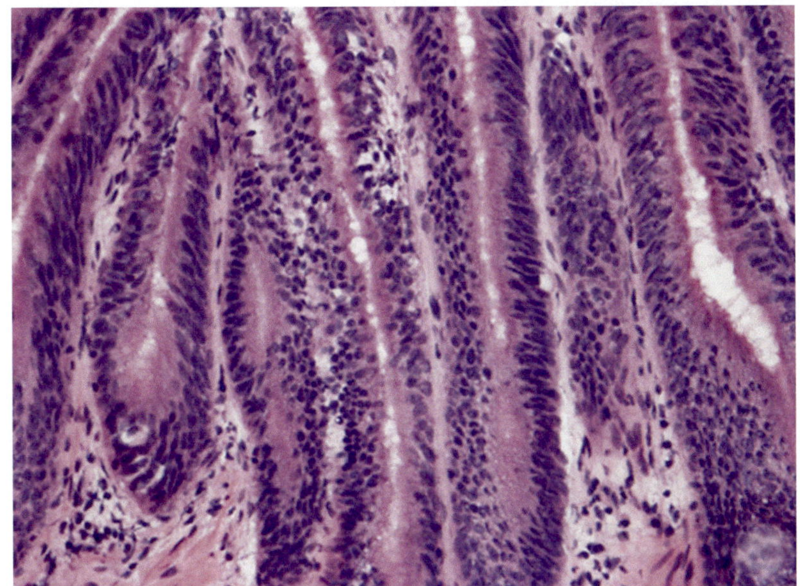

FIG. 6.27 The tubular glands of this ampullary adenoma show low-grade dysplasia. The nuclei are hyperchromatic and elongated with pseudostratification. The cells maintain their polarity and complex architectural features are lacking.

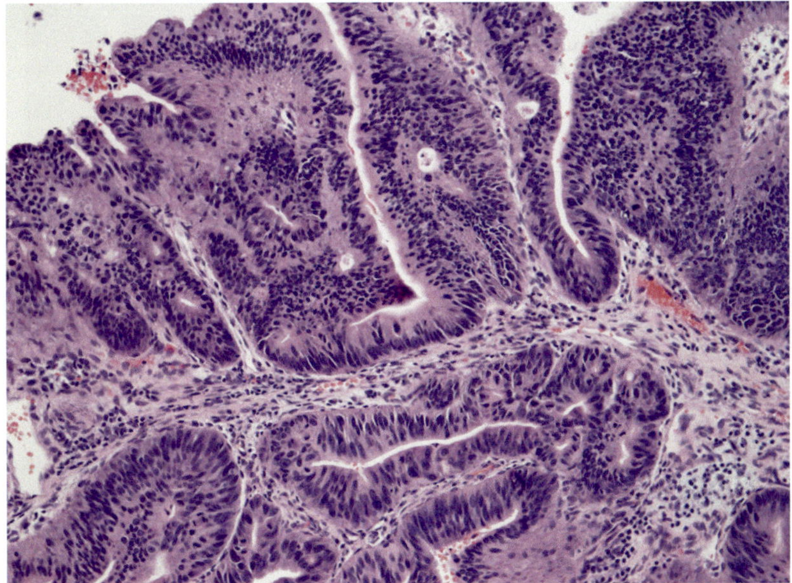

FIG. 6.28 This ampullary adenoma with high-grade dysplasia contains neoplastic glands with a cribriform architecture. The cells show loss of polarity, numerous mitotic figures, and abundant apoptotic debris.

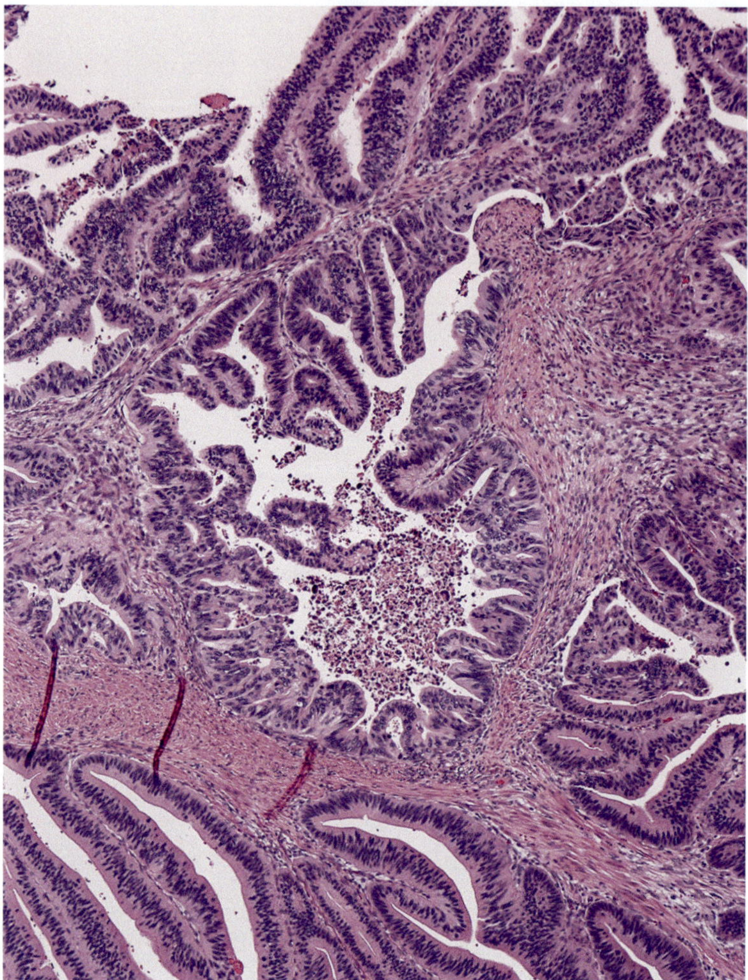

FIG. 6.29 Intestinal-type ampullary adenocarcinomas contain malignant glands with cribriform architecture and luminal necrotic debris, similar to their colonic counterparts. The surrounding stroma is desmoplastic.

of lamina propria, rather than the desmoplastic stroma typical of invasive carcinomas [30]. Instrumentation and repeat biopsies of the ampulla also induce reparative epithelial cell changes that simulate features of adenocarcinoma. Reactive epithelial cell atypia in non-neoplastic epithelium mimics dysplasia and cancer, particularly when mucosal erosions are present (Figs. 6.33 and 6.34). Reactive ampullary glands show nuclear enlargement and macronucleoli, but the nuclei are smooth and round with evenly dispersed chromatin. Cytologic atypia is generally more pronounced in deeper glands, which show surface maturation (Fig. 6.35).

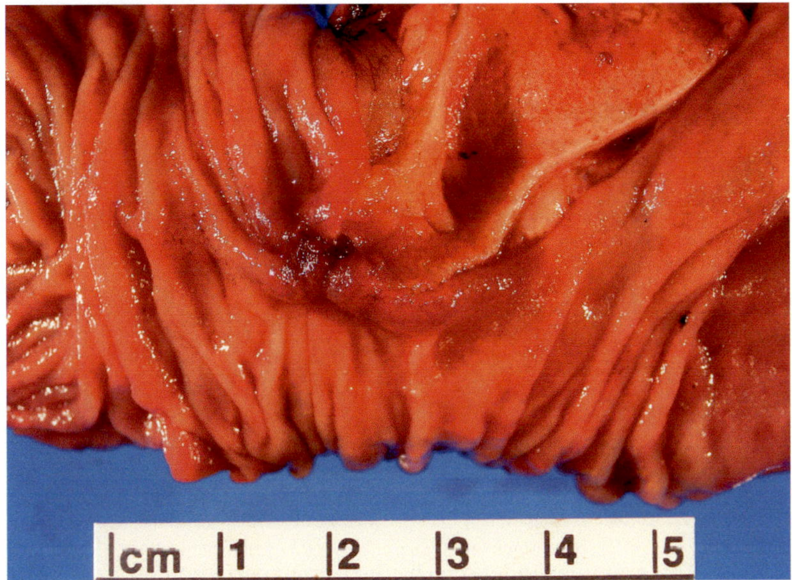

Fɪɢ. 6.30 This adenocarcinoma caused a stricture at the ampulla. The ampullary mucosa is nodular and erythematous.

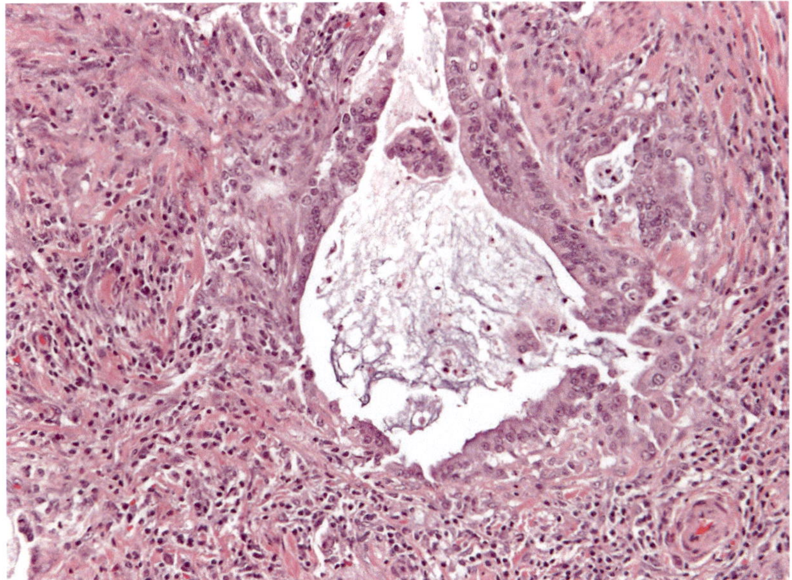

Fɪɢ. 6.31 Pancreatobiliary-type ampullary adenocarcinoma contains mucin-producing, irregularly shaped glands within desmoplastic stroma.

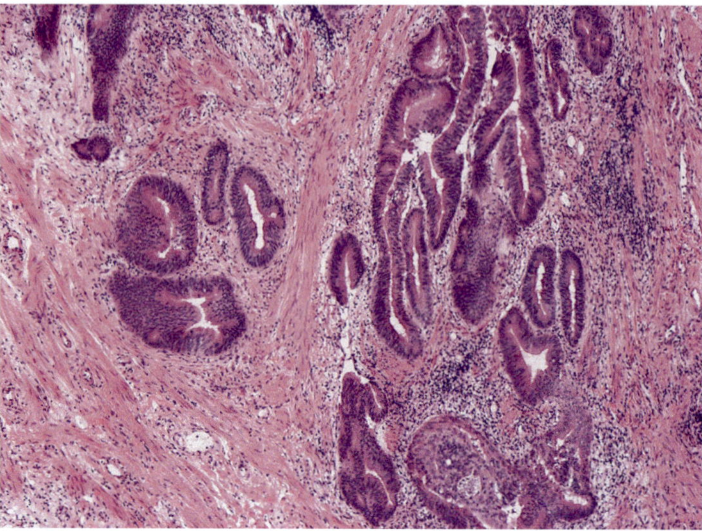

Fig. 6.32   This ampullary adenoma has colonized periampullary glands that are surrounded by smooth muscle bundles, thereby simulating carcinoma. Features that suggest a benign diagnosis include the well-circumscribed appearance of this aggregate, a rim of lamina propria around glands, and the low-grade cytologic appearance of the lesional cells, which are similar to those of the overlying adenoma.

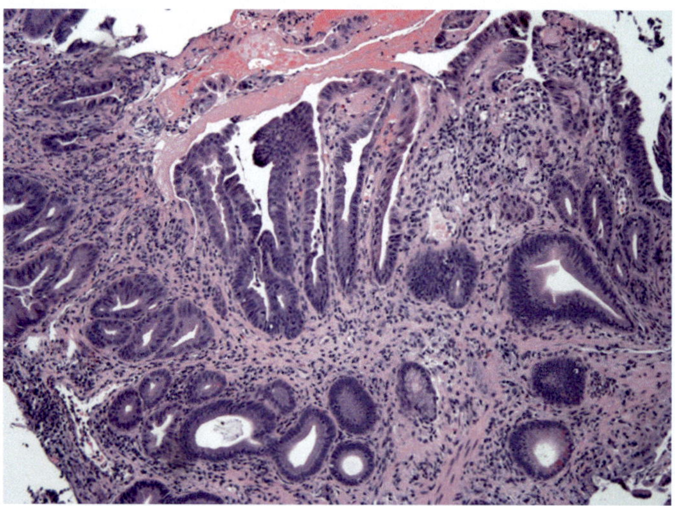

Fig. 6.33   This ampullary biopsy contains a mucosal erosion. The surface is partially denuded with fibrin and inflammatory cells. Adjacent epithelial cells are mucin depleted with large nuclei. The biopsy was taken from a patient with a common bile duct stent.

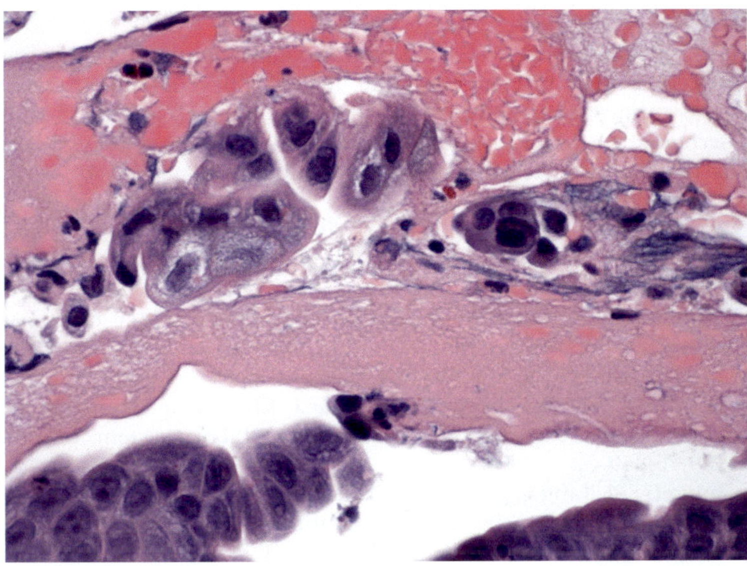

F_{IG}. 6.34 Sloughed epithelial cells show nuclear enlargement and hyperchromasia with irregular contours. However, they still contain abundant cytoplasm and are similar to benign cells in the intact mucosa below (same case as Fig. 6.33).

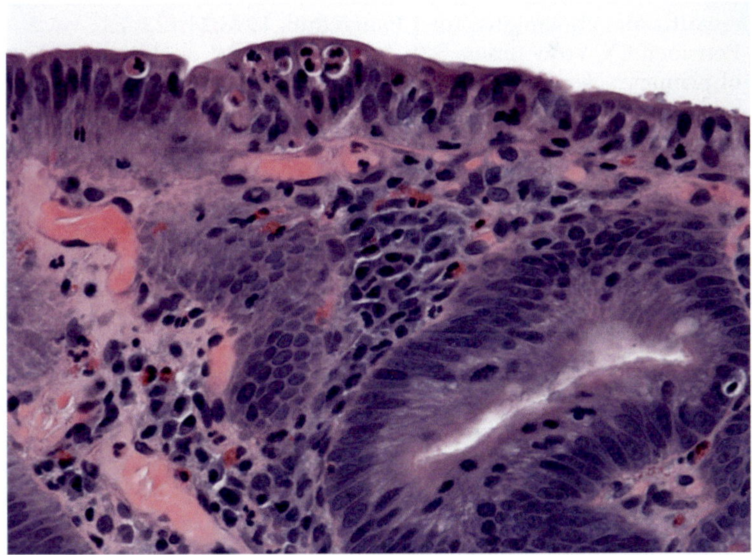

F_{IG}. 6.35 Reactive ampullary glands contain cells with enlarged hyperchromatic nuclei that mimic neoplasia. However, surface maturation and intraepithelial neutrophils are present.

References

1. Binkley CE, Eckhauser FE, Colletti LM. Unusual causes of benign biliary strictures with cholangiographic features of cholangiocarcinoma. J Gastrointest Surg. 2002;6:676–81.
2. Gerhards MF, Vos P, van Gulik TM, et al. Incidence of benign lesions in patients resected for suspicious hilar obstruction. Br J Surg. 2001;88:48–51.
3. Verbeek PC, van Leeuwen DJ, de Wit LT, et al. Benign fibrosing disease at the hepatic confluence mimicking Klatskin tumors. Surgery. 1992;112:866–71.
4. Wetter LA, Ring EJ, Pellegrini CA, Way LW. Differential diagnosis of sclerosing cholangiocarcinomas of the common hepatic duct (Klatskin tumors). Am J Surg. 1991;161:57–62.
5. Standfield NJ, Salisbury JR, Howard ER. Benign non-traumatic inflammatory strictures of the extrahepatic biliary system. Br J Surg. 1989;76:849–52.
6. Chung DTM, Tang CN, Lai ECH, Yang GPC, Li MKW. Immunoglobulin G4-associated sclerosing cholangitis mimicking cholangiocarcinoma. Hong Kong Med J. 2010;16:149–52.
7. Lillemoe KD, Pitt HA, Cameron JL. Postoperative bile duct strictures. Surg Clin North Am. 1990;70:1355–80.
8. Raju GS. Postoperative bile duct strictures. Curr Treat Options Gastroenterol. 2002;5(2):113–21.
9. Charatcharoenwitthaya P, Lindor KD. Primary sclerosing cholangitis: diagnosis and management. Curr Gastroenterol Rep. 2006;8:75–82.
10. Kazumori H, Ashizawa N, Moriyama N, et al. Primary sclerosing pancreatitis and cholangitis. Int J Pancreatol. 1998;24:123–7.
11. Ponsioen CY, Vrouenraets SM, Prawirodirdjo W, et al. Natural history of primary sclerosing cholangitis and prognostic value of cholangiography in a Dutch population. Gut. 2002;51:562–6.
12. Bergquist A, Ekbom A, Olsson R, et al. Hepatic and extrahepatic malignancies in primary sclerosing cholangitis. J Hepatol. 2002;36:321–7.
13. Okazaki K, Uchida K, Ohana M, et al. Autoimmune-related pancreatitis is associated with autoantibodies and a Th1/Th2 – type cellular immune response. Gastroenterol. 2000;118:573–81.
14. Hamano H, Kawa S, Horiuchi A, et al. High serum IgG4 concentrations in patients with sclerosing pancreatitis. N Engl J Med. 2001;344:732–8.
15. Ghazale A, Chari ST, Zhang L, et al. Immunoglobulin G4-associated cholangitis: clinical profile and response to therapy. Gastroenterology. 2008;134:706–15.
16. Zhang L, Smyrk TC. Autoimmune pancreatitis and IgG4-related systemic diseases. Int J Clin Exp Pathol. 2010;3(5):491–504.
17. Kawakami H, Zen Y, Kuwatani M, et al. IgG4-related sclerosing cholangitis and autoimmune pancreatitis: histological assessment of biopsies from Vater's ampulla and the bile duct. J Gastroenterol Hepatol. 2010;25:1648–55.
18. Liu YB, Wang JW, Devkota KR, et al. Congenital choledochal cysts in adults: twenty-five year experience. Chin Med J. 2007;120(16):1404–7.

19. Todani T, Watanabe Y, Narusue M, Tabuchi K, Okajima K. Congenital bile duct cysts. Classification, operative procedures, a review of thirty-seven cases including cancer arising from a choledochal cyst. Am J Surg. 1977;134:263–9.
20. Chijiiwa K, Koga A. Surgical management and long-term follow-up of patients with choledochal cysts. Am J Surg. 1993;165:238–42.
21. Liu CL, Fan ST, Lo CM, et al. Choledochal cysts in adults. Arch Surg. 2002;137:465–8.
22. Albores-Saavedra J, Adsay NV, Crawford JM, et al. Tumours of the gallbladder and extrahepatic biliary tree. In: Bosman FT, Carneiro F, Hruban RH, Theise ND, editors. WHO classification of tumours of the digestive system. 4th ed. Lyon: IARC Press; 2010. p. 263–76.
23. Meza-Junco J, Montano-Loza AJ, Ma M, Wong W, Sawyer MB, Bain VG. Cholangiocarcinoma: has there been any progress? Can J Gastroenterol. 2010;24(1):52–7.
24. Sakamoto Y, Shimada K, Nara S, et al. Surgical management of infrahilar/suprapancreatic cholangiocarcinoma: an analysis of the surgical procedures, surgical margins, and survivals of 77 patients. J Gastrointest Surg. 2010;14(2):335–43.
25. Adsay NV, Klimstra DS. Benign and malignant tumors of the gallbladder and extrahepatic biliary tree. In: Odze RD, Goldblum JR, editors. Surgical pathology of the GI tract, liver, biliary tract, and pancreas. 2nd ed. Philadelphia: Saunders Elsevier; 2009. p. 845–75.
26. Konishi M, Iwasaki M, Ochiai A, Hasebe T, Ojima H, Yanagisawa A. Clinical impact of intraoperative histologic examination of the ductal resection margin in extrahepatic cholangiocarcinoma. Br J Surg. 2010;97(9):1363–8.
27. Achille A, Baron A, Zamboni G, Di Pace C, Orlandini S, Scarpa A. Chromosome 5 allelic losses are early in tumours of the papilla of Vater and occur at sites similar to those of gastric cancer. Br J Cancer. 1998;78(12):1653–60.
28. Heinrich S, Clavien P-A. Ampullary cancer. Curr Opin Gastroenterol. 2010;26(3):280–5.
29. Wong RF, DiSario JA. Approaches to endoscopic ampullectomy. Curr Opin Gastroenterol. 2004;20(5):460–7.
30. Yantiss RK, Antonioli DA. Polyps of the small intestine. In: Odze RD, Goldblum JR, editors. Surgical pathology of the GI tract, liver, biliary tract, and pancreas. 2nd ed. Philadelphia: Saunders Elsevier; 2009. p. 447–80.

Chapter 7
Intraoperative Evaluation of the Gallbladder

INTRODUCTION

Only 0.35% of gallbladder adenocarcinomas are incidentally discovered during surgical exploration for cholecystitis, but surgeons who encounter a contracted, thickened, or discolored gallbladder may request frozen section consultation to rule out the possibility of adenocarcinoma [1]. Several nonneoplastic conditions that simulate gallbladder neoplasia are encountered by pathologists at frozen section analysis, which has a high sensitivity and specificity for distinguishing benign from malignant conditions [2, 3].

NONNEOPLASTIC MIMICS OF GALLBLADDER CARCINOMA
Cholesterol Polyps and Cholesterolosis

Cholesterol polyps are encountered in 4–8% of patients undergoing cholecystectomy [4]. These benign mucosal lesions result from localized accumulations of macrophages that contain cholesterol esters and triglycerides. Cholesterol polyps are correctly classified by ultrasonographic evaluation in most cases, but those larger than 1 cm in diameter raise concern for malignancy and may be evaluated intraoperatively [5]. Cholesterol polyps are smooth yellow-to-white mucosa-based nodules consisting of collections of lipid-laden macrophages (Figs. 7.1 and 7.2). They may be associated with a more diffuse accumulation of lipid-laden macrophages in the mucosa, termed cholesterolosis (Fig. 7.3) [6].

Xanthogranulomatous Cholecystitis

Xanthogranulomatous cholecystitis is a form of chronic cholecystitis that causes tumor-like thickening of the gallbladder wall

R.K. Yantiss (ed.), *Frozen Section Library: Liver, Extrahepatic Biliary Tree and Gallbladder*, Frozen Section Library, DOI 10.1007/978-1-4614-0043-1_7,
© Springer Science+Business Media, LLC 2011

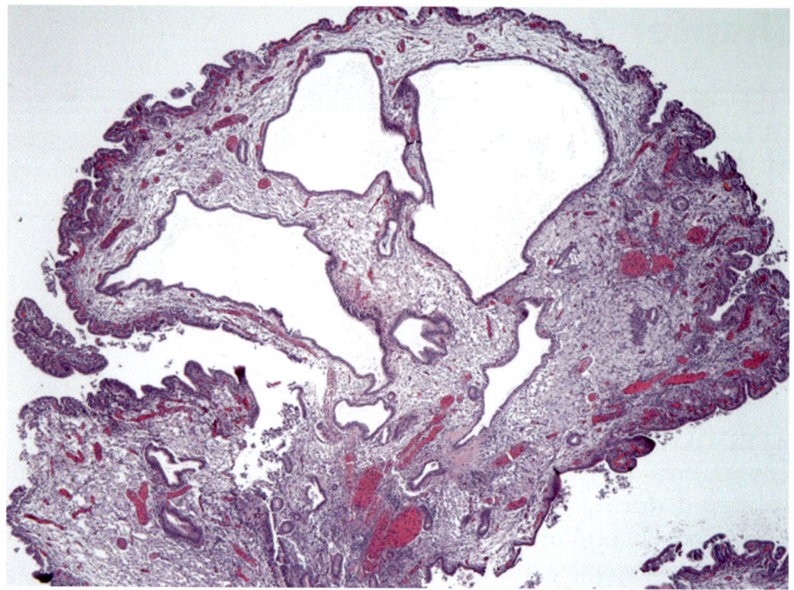

FIG. 7.1 Cholesterol polyps are smooth, muscosa-based nodules comprised of macrophages. This one also contains numerous cysts lined by benign epithelium.

and may involve adjacent structures, such as the liver, colon, small intestine, and abdominal wall (Fig. 7.4) [7, 8]. Inflammatory changes obscure tissue planes and simulate the appearance of a malignancy, so this finding at cholecystectomy may prompt intraoperative consultation. Xanthogranulomatous cholecystitis reflects an exuberant inflammatory response to ruptured Rokitansky-Aschoff sinuses and extrusion of bile and cholesterol into the gallbladder wall. Extraluminal bile elicits a macrophage-rich inflammatory response (Figs. 7.5 and 7.6). Xanthogranulomatous areas are yellow, reflecting the presence of collections of lipid-laden macrophages and cholesterol clefts admixed with giant cells, acute and chronic inflammation, and extensive fibrosis (Figs. 7.7 and 7.8) [9].

Aberrant (Luschka's) Ducts

Aberrant (Luschka's) ducts are small biliary-type ductules that are commonly found in the hepatic bed or, less frequently, the subserosal connective tissue of the gallbladder. They occur in small clusters surrounded by a thin rim of loose cellular stroma and contain epithelial cells resembling those of intrahepatic bile ducts (Fig. 7.9). Their location outside the gallbladder wall can cause confusion with invasive adenocarcinoma, particularly when associated with adjacent hepatic parenchyma. Aberrant ducts show florid

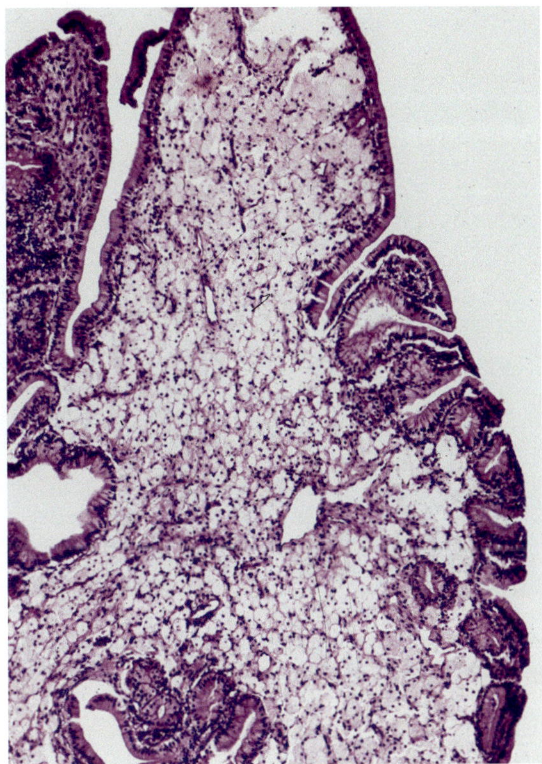

FIG. 7.2 Cholesterol polyps contain numerous lipid-laden macrophages that fill the lamina propria.

hyperplasia in patients with acute cholecystitis and serositis. In this situation, the proliferating ductules are arranged in linear arrays along the gallbladder fossa and within the subserosa (Fig. 7.10). The ducts may show slight cytologic atypia, but the nuclei are smooth and round without mitotic activity (Fig. 7.11) [9].

Rokitansky-Aschoff Sinuses

Rokitansky-Aschoff sinuses are acquired pseudodiverticula of the gallbladder that are frequently found in patients with chronic cholecystitis and probably result from repetitive contraction of the gallbladder against outflow obstruction due to cholelithiasis. Rokitansky-Aschoff sinuses are located within the muscularis propria, although they may protrude into the connective tissue outside the gallbladder wall, and contain a biliary epithelial cell lining, similar to that of the overlying mucosa (Figs. 7.12 and 7.13). They are oriented perpendicularly to the gallbladder lumen and often communicate with the mucosal surface. The distinction between

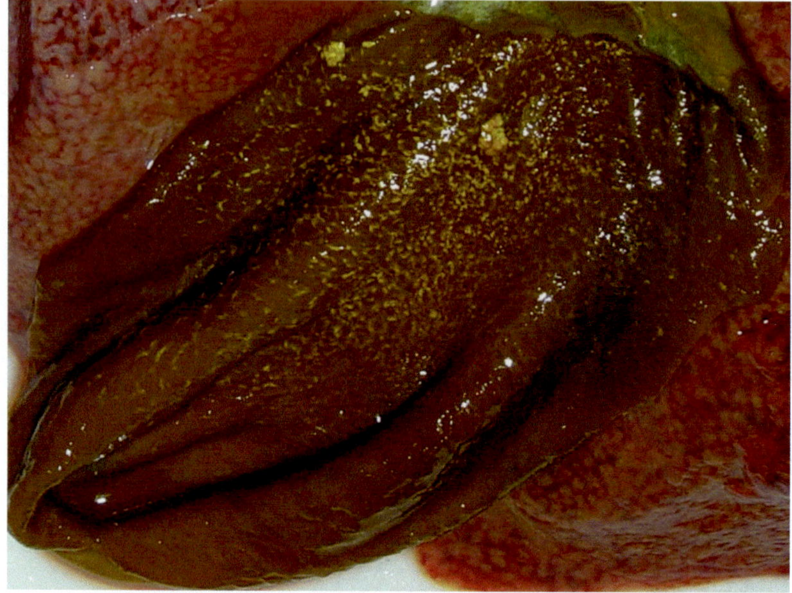

FIG. 7.3 Diffuse cholesterolosis imparts a gold-flecked appearance to the mucosa owing to aggregates of macrophages in the lamina propria.

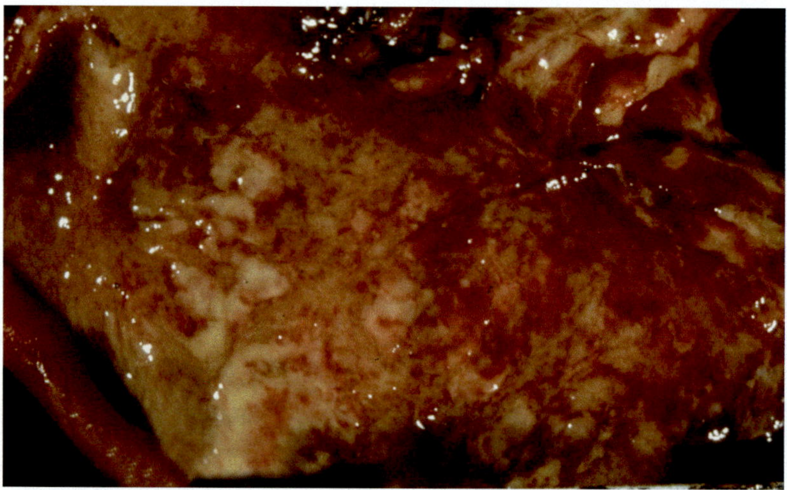

FIG. 7.4 Xanthogranulomatous inflammation in the gallbladder produces thickened and nodular areas in the wall with yellow discoloration.

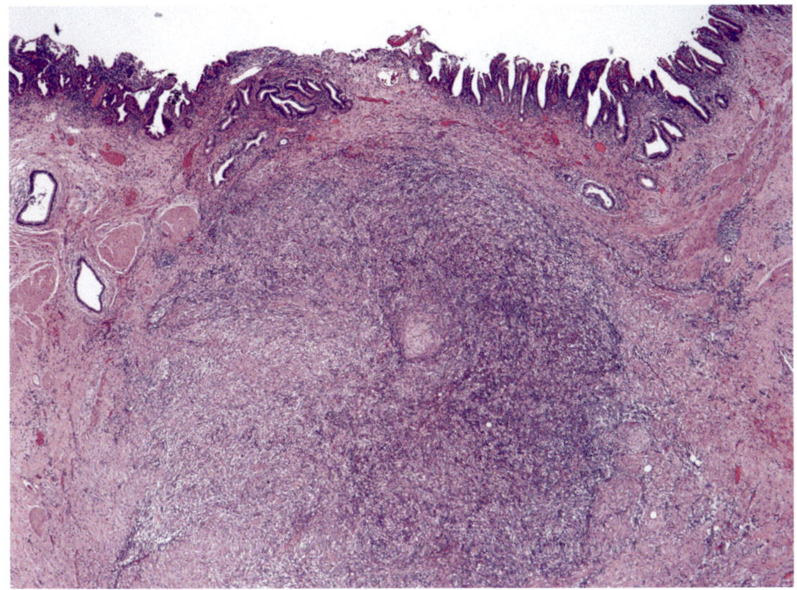

FIG. 7.5 Xanthogranulomatous inflammation obliterates a ruptured Rokitansky-Aschoff sinus in the gallbladder wall.

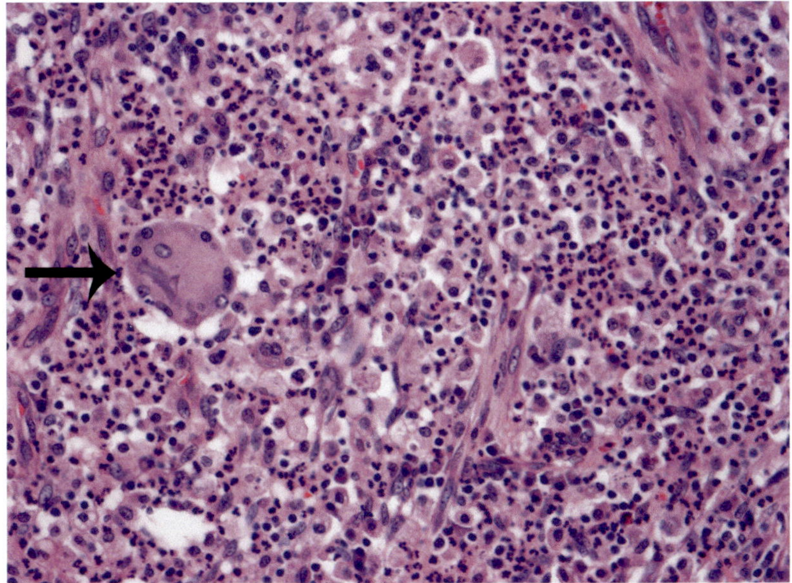

FIG. 7.6 The inflammatory infiltrate of xanthogranulomatous cholecystitis consists of mononuclear cells and scattered giant cells (*arrow*).

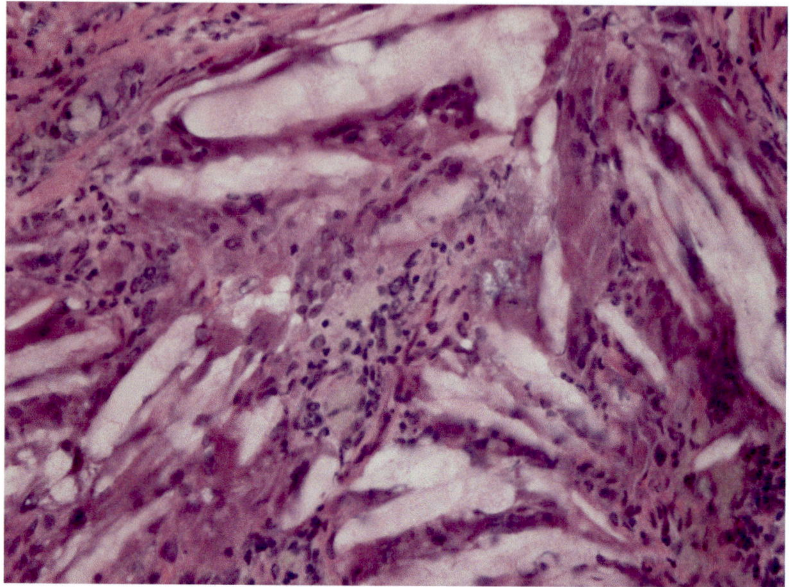

FIG. 7.7 Cholesterol clefts surrounded by giant cells are apparent in this case of xanthogranulomatous cholecystitis.

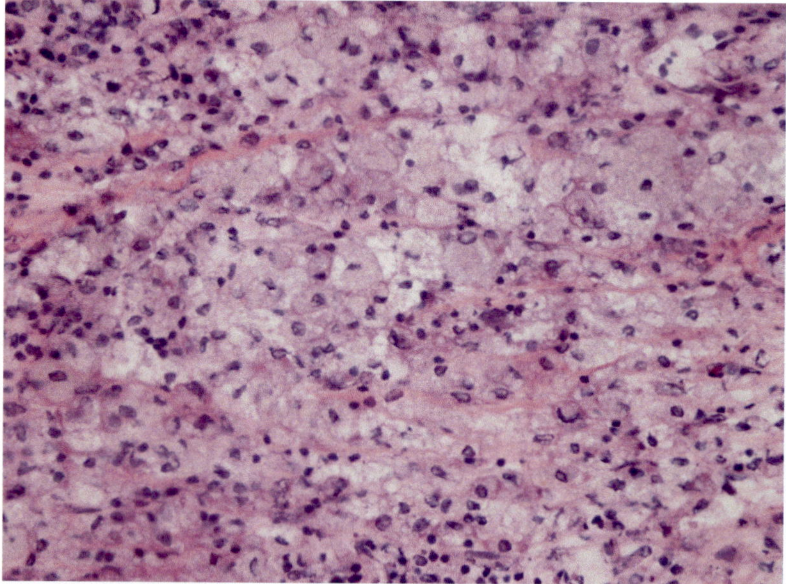

FIG. 7.8 Aggregates of lipid-rich macrophages are characteristic of xanthogranulomatous cholecystitis.

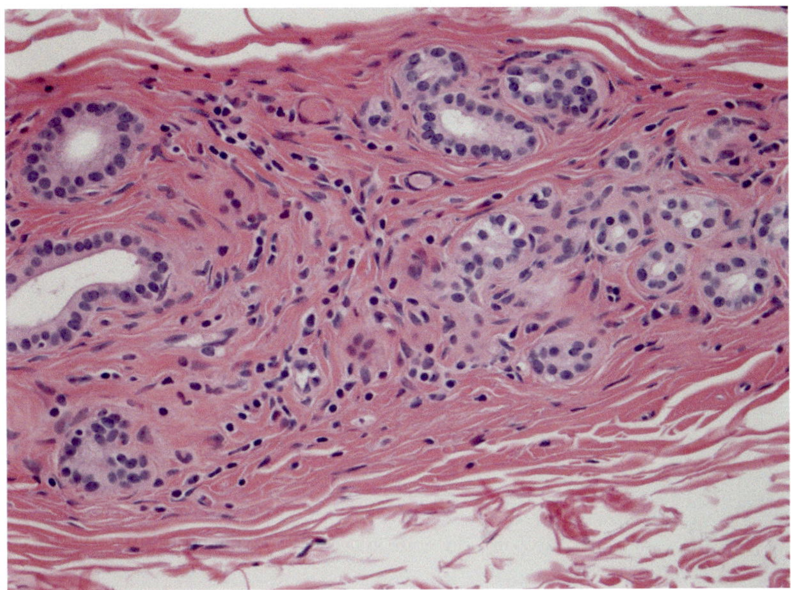

FIG. 7.9 Aberrant (Luschka's) ducts are commonly identified in gallbladders with serositis and cholecystitis. Small clusters of bile ductules are present within inflammatory stroma.

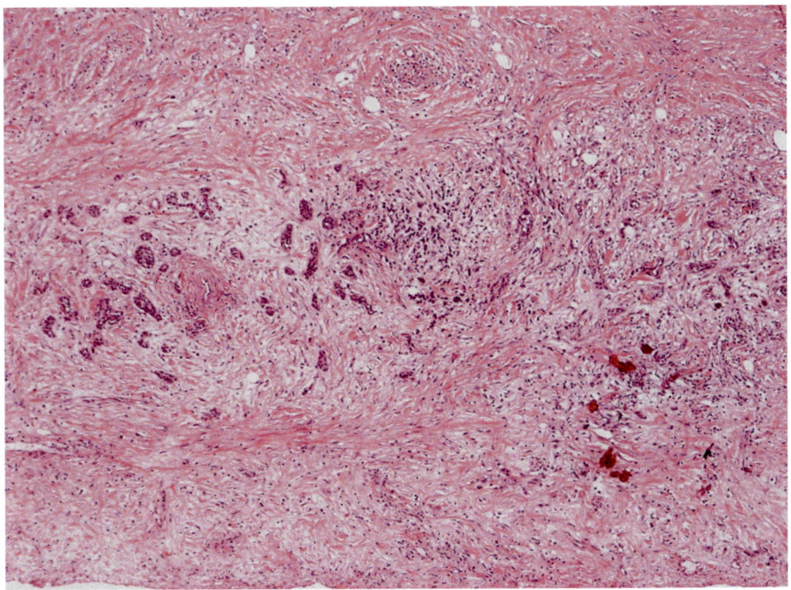

FIG. 7.10 Florid aberrant (Luschka's) ducts show a linear proliferation of small tubules best appreciated at low magnification.

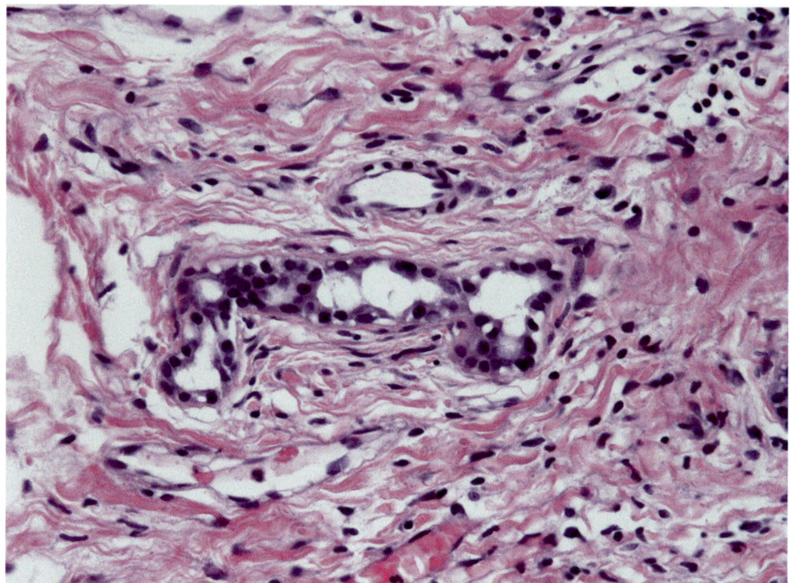

FIG. 7.11 Aberrant (Luschka's) ducts contain cuboidal cells with basally located nuclei that resemble benign biliary ducts and show minimal, if any, cytologic atypia.

prominent Rokitansky-Aschoff sinuses and invasive adenocarcinoma is usually straightforward, but colonization by dysplasia and inflammation-induced reactive epithelial changes may mimic carcinoma in rare cases, particularly when confounded by frozen section artifacts. Extensive branching of Rokitansky-Aschoff sinuses produces tubules oriented parallel to the lumen (Fig. 7.14) [10, 11]. Rokitansky-Achoff sinuses may also become dilated and rupture, leading to accumulation of extruded mucin in the wall. Some mucin pools contain detached fragments of biliary epithelium, simulating adenocarcinoma (Fig. 7.15). Ruptured diverticula elicit a fibroinflammatory stromal response that resembles the desmoplastic stroma of carcinoma (Fig. 7.16). In this situation, it is helpful to remember that mucinous adenocarcinomas of the gallbladder are rare and, when present, are accompanied by a component of conventional adenocarcinoma [10]. Disrupted Rokitansky-Aschoff sinuses may also show displaced epithelium adjacent to nerves that closely approximates the appearance of perineural invasion by carcinoma (Fig. 7.17) [11]. A summary of the features that aid distinction between Rokitansky-Achoff sinuses and adenocarcinoma is presented in Table 7.1.

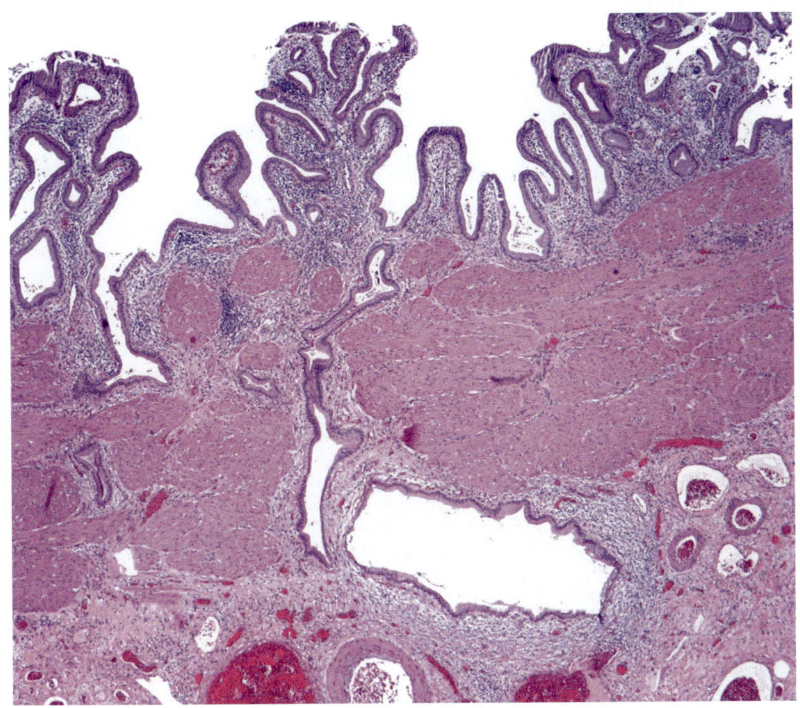

FIG. 7.12 Rokitansky-Aschoff sinuses represent herniations of mucosa into, or through, the muscularis propria.

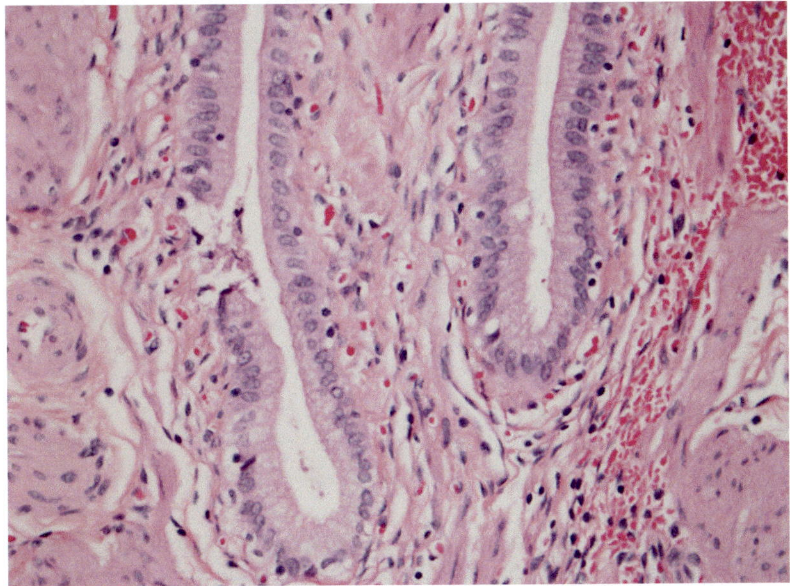

FIG. 7.13 Rokitansky-Aschoff sinuses are lined by benign cuboidal biliary epithelium with basally located nuclei.

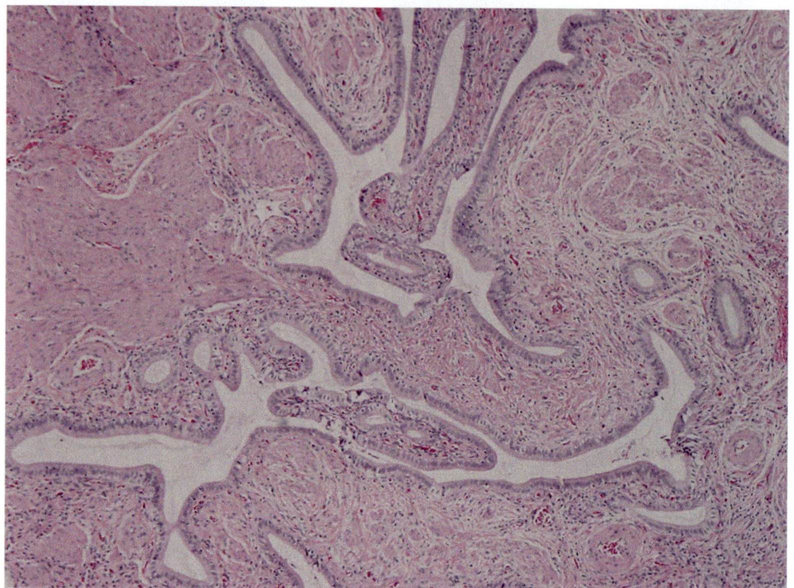

Fɪɢ. 7.14 Branching of Rokitansky-Aschoff sinuses appear as laterally branched glands oriented parallel to the gallbladder lumen.

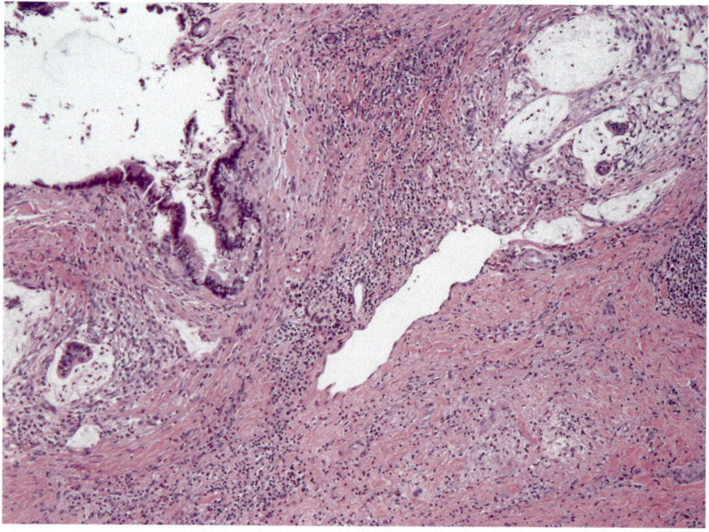

Fɪɢ. 7.15 A ruptured Rokitansky-Aschoff sinus is dilated and partially denuded. Fibroinflammatory stroma surrounds mucin pools in the gallbladder wall (photograph courtesy of Dr. David Klimstra, Memorial Sloan-Kettering cancer Center).

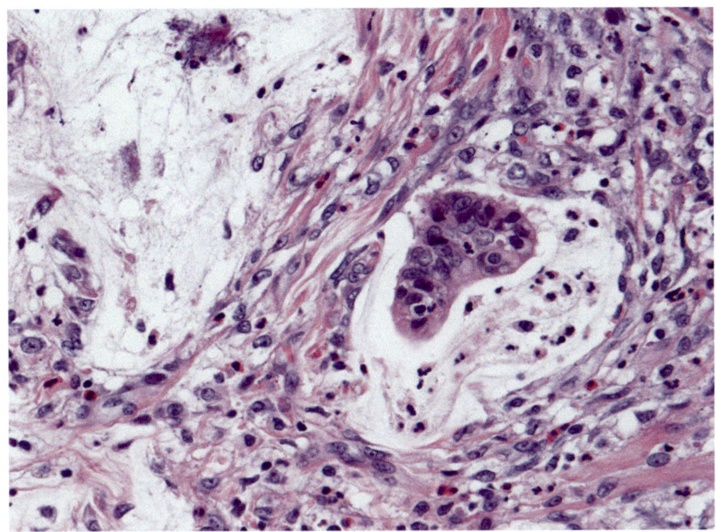

FIG. 7.16 A ruptured Rokitansky-Aschoff sinus is associated with mural mucin pools. The pools are surrounded by inflammatory stroma. They contain nonneoplastic inflammatory cells that simulate mucinous carcinoma (photograph courtesy of Dr. David Klimstra, Memorial Sloan-Kettering cancer Center).

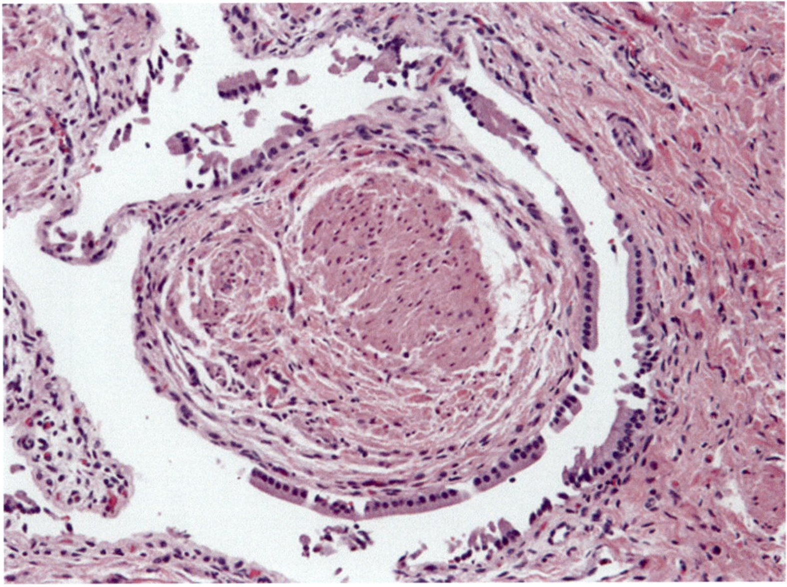

FIG. 7.17 A ruptured Rokitansky-Aschoff sinus is associated with displaced epithelium in close proximity to a nerve, simulating perineural invasion of invasive adenocarcinoma (photograph courtesy of Dr. David Klimstra, Memorial-Sloan Kettering Cancer Center).

TABLE 7.1   Distinguishing features of benign biliary lesions and gallbladder adenocarcinoma.

Feature	Aberrant ducts (of Luschka)	Rokitansky-Aschoff sinuses	Adenomyosis	Adenocarcinoma
Gross appearance	Cholecystitis	Cholecystitis Mural cysts	Mural nodularity Mural cysts	Ill-defined mass Polyp
Pathologic features				
Epithelial orientation	Well-circumscribed linear proliferation of small ductules in hepatic bed or serosa	Well-circumscribed mural cysts oriented perpendicular to lumen	Well-circumscribed proliferation of small glands and cysts perpendicular to lumen	Haphazard proliferation of irregular glands parallel to lumen
Communication with lumen	Absent	Present	Absent	Absent
Extruded mucin	Absent	Occasionally present Rarely contains nonneoplastic epithelium	Absent	Occasionally present May contain neoplastic epithelium
Glandular morphology	Small round ductules	Cystic glands	Cysts and small ductules	Angulated glands
	Cytologically bland	Cytologically bland	Cytologically bland	Cytologically malignant

Adenomyoma and Adenomyomatous Hyperplasia

Hypertrophy and hyperplasia of smooth muscle cells adjacent to Rokitansky-Aschoff sinuses results in diffuse, or localized, thickening of the gallbladder wall, termed adenomyomatous hyperplasia, or adenomyoma, respectively [6]. Adenomyomatous hyperplasia produces grossly evident cystically dilated mural spaces, whereas adenomyomas are variably solid and cystic depending on the relative amounts of biliary mucosa and smooth muscle in the lesion (Fig. 7.18). The cysts are lined by benign biliary epithelium and surrounded by hypertrophic smooth muscle bundles (Figs. 7.19 and 7.20). Some adenomyomas contain proliferating small ductules enmeshed in smooth muscle (Fig. 7.21). Perineural and intraneural epithelium is a well-described phenomenon seen

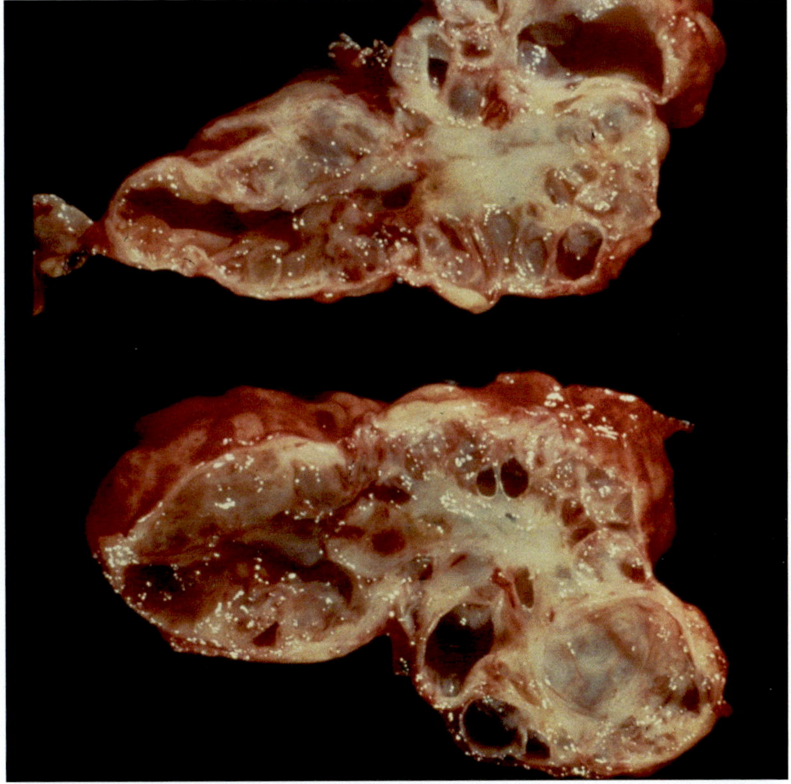

FIG. 7.18 Adenomyomatous hyperplasia produces innumerable cysts in the gallbladder wall.

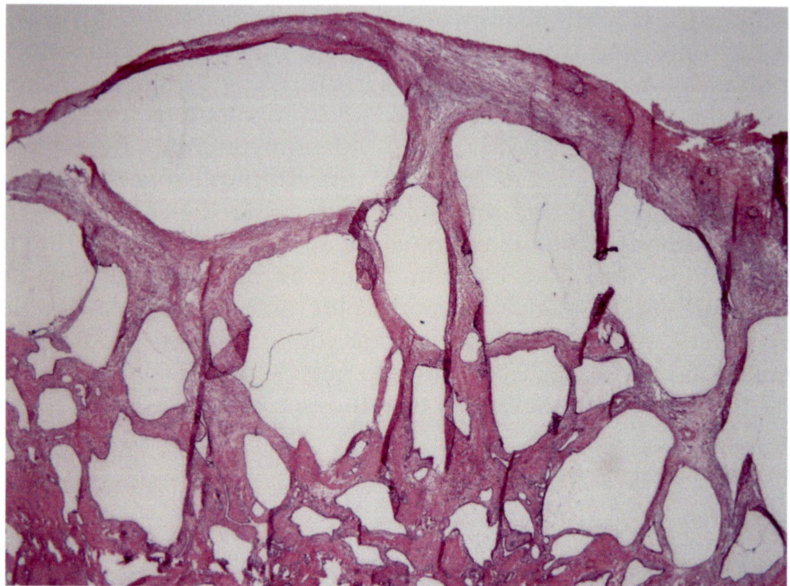

FIG. 7.19 An adenomyoma contains numerous cysts, each of which is surrounded by a concentric proliferation of smooth muscle cells.

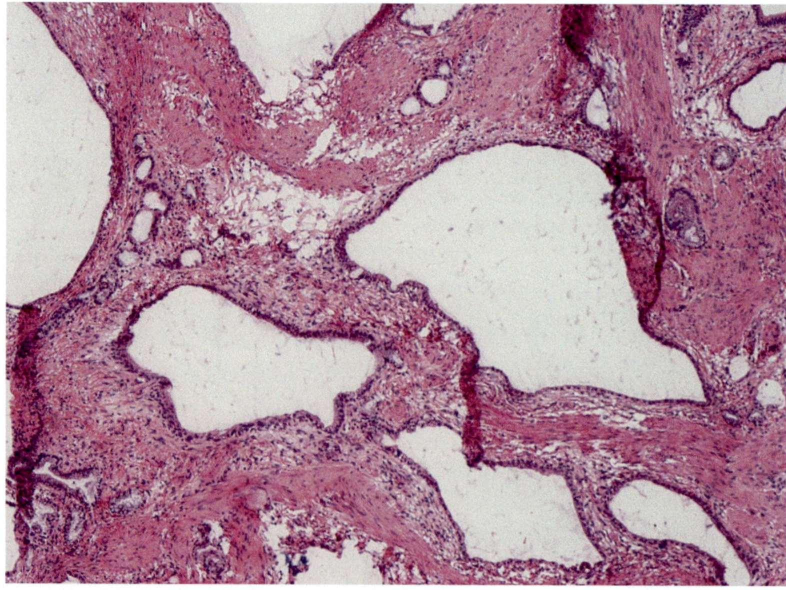

FIG. 7.20 The cysts of an adenomyoma are lined by cytologically bland, nonneoplastic biliary-type epithelium.

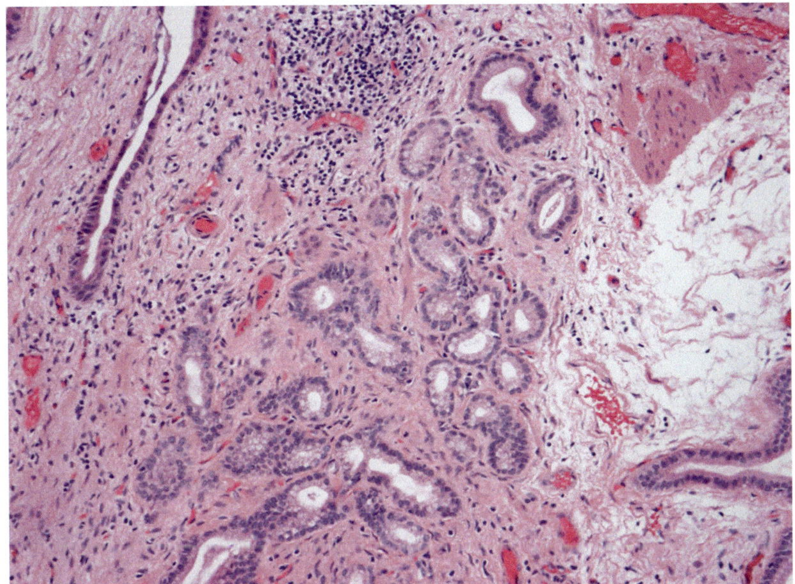

FIG. 7.21 Some adenomyomas contain smaller proliferating ductules as well as cysts.

in adenomyomatous hyperplasia [11]. This finding should not be interpreted to represent malignancy in the absence of cytologic features of carcinoma.

BENIGN GALLBLADDER NEOPLASMS THAT PRODUCE POLYPS

Gallbladder adenomas display a spectrum of morphologic features and are classified as pyloric gland-, intestinal-, and biliary-type adenomas [6]. Pyloric gland adenomas are most common. They are composed of tightly packed glands with little intervening stroma (Fig. 7.22). The cells contain abundant neutral mucin and round, regular, basally located nuclei, resembling duodenal Brunner's glands, or gastric glands in the pyloric region (Fig. 7.23). They may also show squamous metaplasia, occasional Paneth cells, or goblet cells. Intestinal-type adenomas resemble colonic adenomas with overt, usually low-grade, dysplasia. Biliary-type adenomas are rare. They contain epithelium resembling that of the normal gallbladder and usually display low-grade cytology (Figs. 7.24 and 7.25). Multifocal gallbladder adenoma, or papillomatosis, is associated with high-grade dysplasia, risk of recurrence, and invasive adenocarcinoma [12].

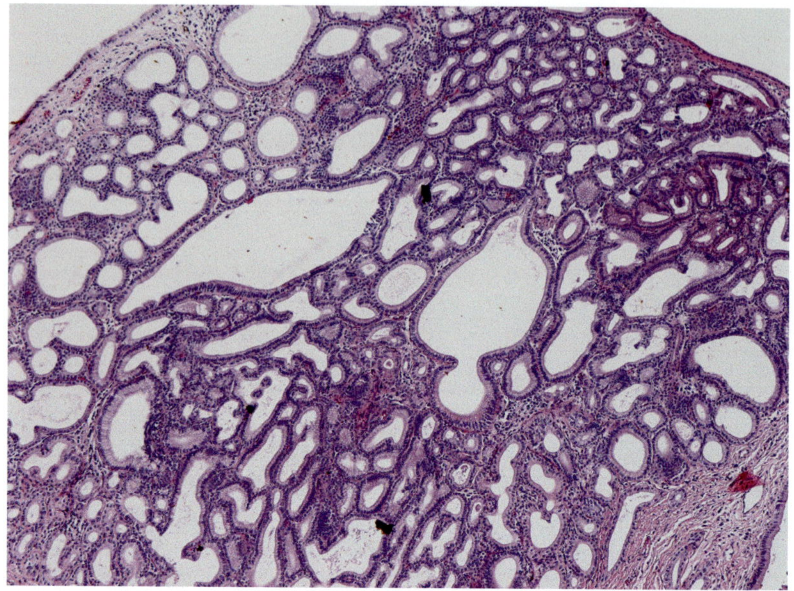

FIG. 7.22 A pyloric gland adenoma contains densely packed, variably cystic glands with little intervening stroma.

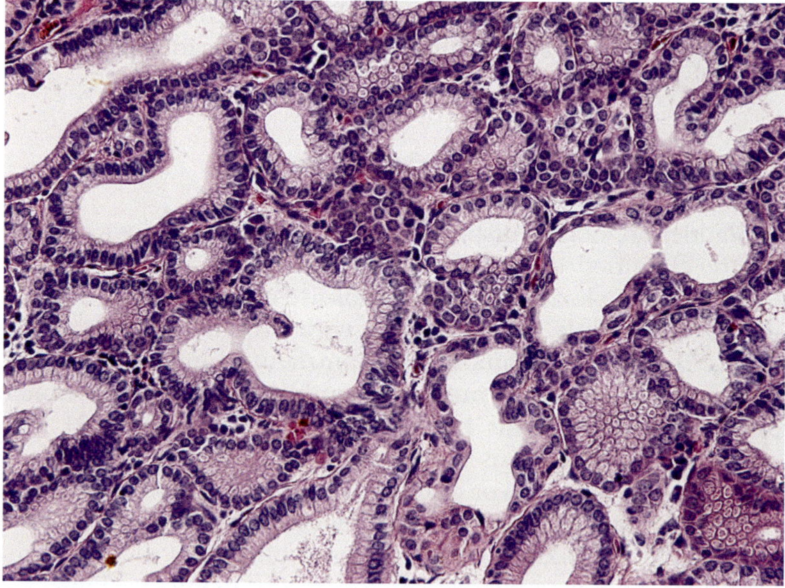

FIG. 7.23 Some of the glands in this pyloric gland adenoma are dilated. They contain polarized, neutral mucin producing epithelial cells with basally located, bland nuclei.

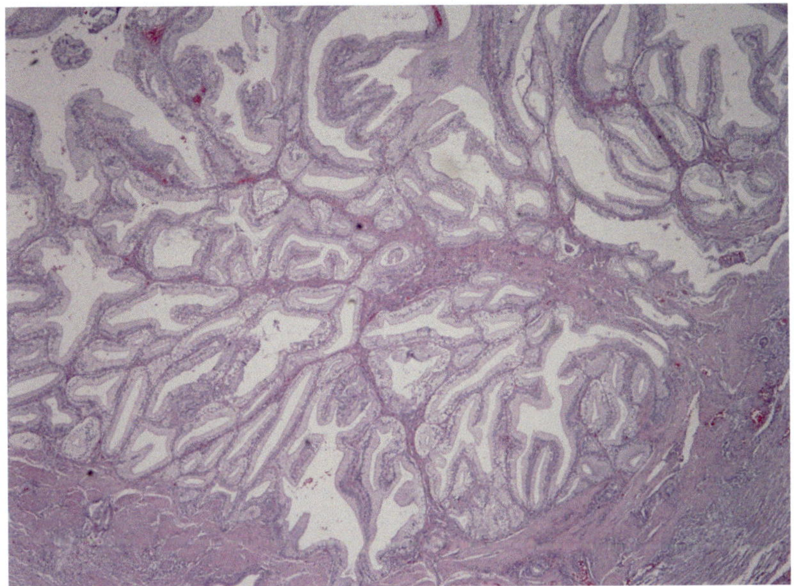

FIG. 7.24 Biliary-type gallbladder adenomas contain well-circumscribed lobules of branching glands with little stroma.

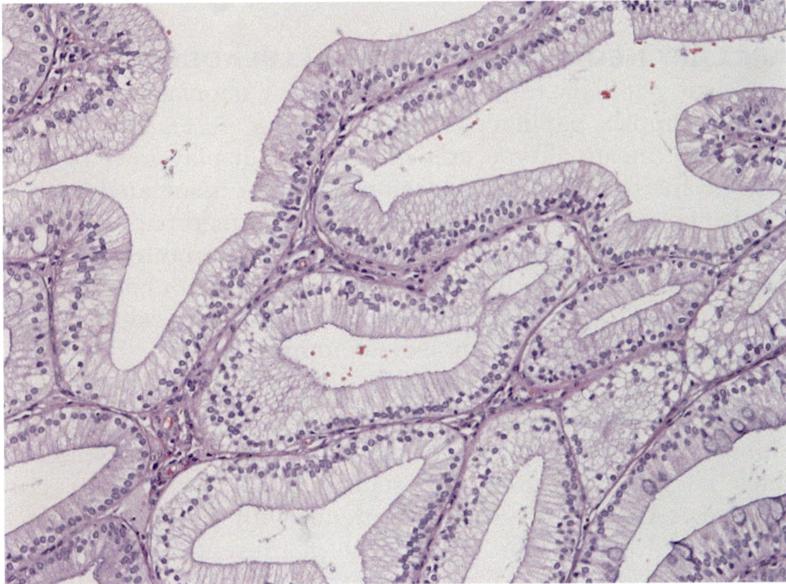

FIG. 7.25 The glands of a biliary-type adenoma contain tall columnar cells with abundant cytoplasm. The nuclei are small, bland, and closely apposed to the basement membrane.

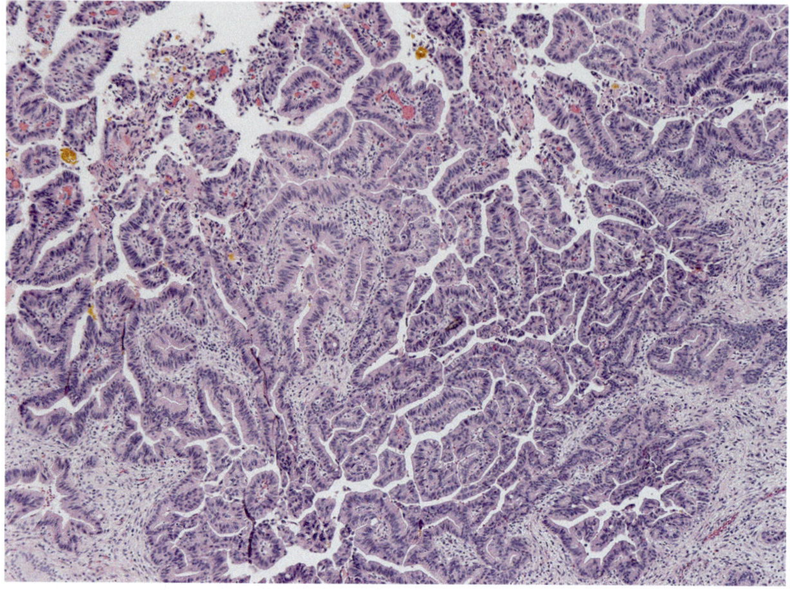

FIG. 7.26 Intracystic papillary neoplasms harbor complex fronds of dysplastic epithelium without intervening stroma.

PAPILLARY NEOPLASMS OF THE GALLBLADDER

Intracystic papillary tumors are preinvasive neoplasms characterized by complex papillary architecture (Fig. 7.26). They contain biliary- or intestinal-type epithelium, and display low- or high-grade dysplasia. High-grade lesions may be associated with an invasive component and, thus, have been termed papillary carcinomas (Fig. 7.27) [12, 13]. The distinction between intracystic papillary neoplasms and gallbladder adenomas may not be possible at the time of frozen section analysis and is not necessary, since all are adequately treated by cholecystectomy.

GALLBLADDER CARCINOMA

Gallbladder carcinoma is an aggressive and lethal disease, for which surgical resection represents the best option for cure. Unfortunately, only 15–40% of patients with gallbladder cancer are eligible for resection at the time of presentation, and those who are operated upon frequently experience disease recurrence despite apparently complete resection [14]. Gallbladder carcinomas are more frequent in patients with long-standing cholelithiasis or an abnormal choledochopancreatic junction. Some older

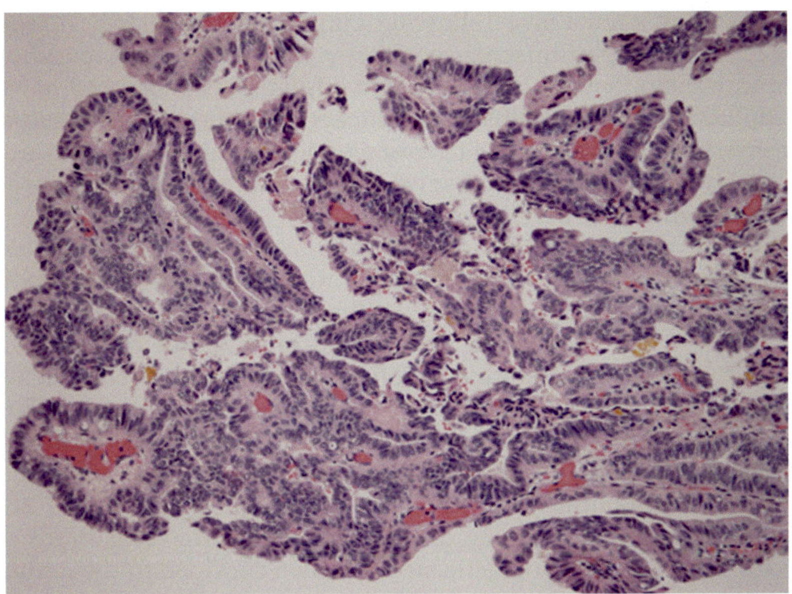

FIG. 7.27   The tumor cells of this intracystic papillary neoplasm are clearly dysplastic. They are cuboidal or columnar with large hyperchromatic nuclei.

data suggest a higher risk for cancer among patients with diffuse calcification of the gallbladder wall (porcelain gallbladder), but more recent data refute this view [15]. Ethnic populations with a high incidence of cholelithiasis, such as Native Americans and those of Latin American descent, also have a higher incidence of gallbladder carcinoma. Patients with familial adenomatous polyposis seem to be at risk for this type of cancer as well [14, 16].

Pathologic tumor stage is the most important determinant of tumor resectability, so pathologists may be asked to evaluate the depth of invasion of gallbladder carcinoma intraoperatively. Carcinomas limited to the lamina propria (T1a) are usually detected in gallbladder adenomas. These early cancers have a risk of lymph node metastasis that is less than 2.5%, so they are adequately treated by simple cholecystectomy [17–20]. Frozen section evaluation of the cystic duct margin may be requested in such cases [21]. Advanced tumors that invade the muscularis propria (T1b) may be similarly treated, or they are managed by radical cholecystectomy with resection of the liver bed [22–24]. Approximately 20% of these cancers are associated with regional lymph node metastases and they frequently display lymphovascular invasion with high risk

(30–60%) of recurrence following cholecystectomy [25]. Tumors that invade the perimuscular connective tissue (T2) require radical cholecystectomy with resection of liver segments IVb/V and portal lymphadenectomy. Gallbladder cancers that perforate the serosa or invade adjacent organs (T3) are diagnosed radiographically and most are not resectable at diagnosis. If possible, resection involves *en bloc* removal of all affected organs [26].

Invasive gallbladder adenocarcinomas appear as polypoid, exophytic masses or diffusely infiltrating tumors. Polypoid tumors are soft and friable, whereas diffusely infiltrative carcinomas are firm, white, and gritty due to the presence of desmoplasia (Fig. 7.28). Most gallbladder adenocarcinomas are histologically similar to pancreatic ductal and bile duct adenocarcinomas. They contain malignant glands associated with desmoplastic stroma (Fig. 7.29). The tumor cells are cuboidal to columnar with neutral mucin-containing cytoplasm and cytologic atypia (Fig. 7.30). Early gallbladder cancers display complex inter-anastomosing glands, but lack desmoplastic stroma when confined to the lamina propria or muscularis propria (Figs. 7.31 and 7.32).

Frozen section analysis of gallbladder cancers is generally limited to three situations: evaluation of the cystic duct margin, assessment of the hepatic bed for adequacy of excision, and

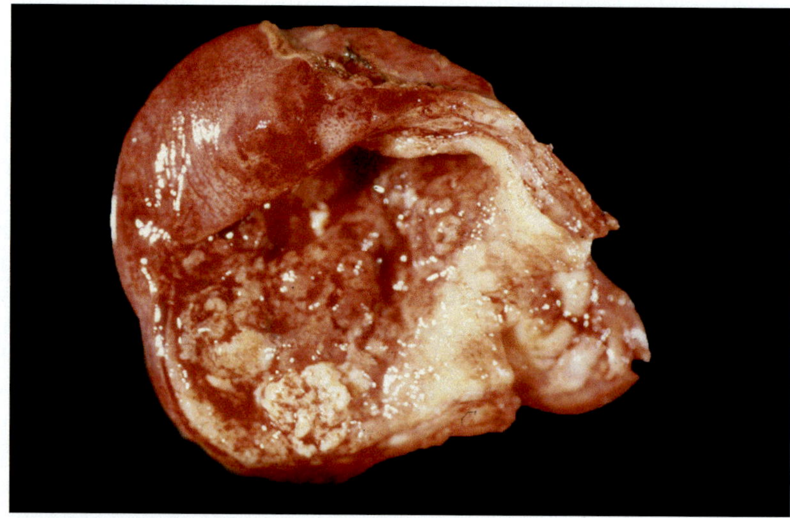

Fig. 7.28 Invasive adenocarcinoma diffusely infiltrates the gallbladder wall and produces multiple mucosal nodules.

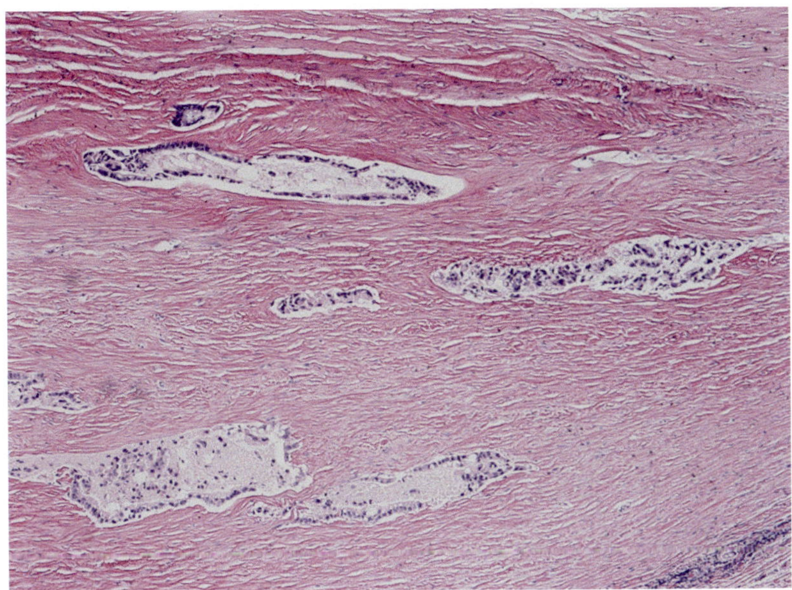

FIG. 7.29 A well-differentiated gallbladder adenocarcinoma is composed of irregular glands within the gallbladder wall. The glands are oriented parallel to the gallbladder lumen. The wall is replaced by collagenous stroma.

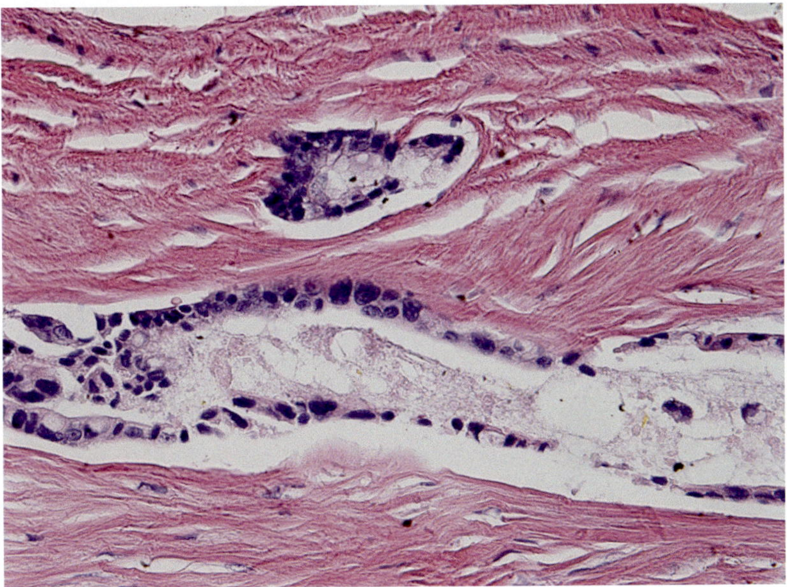

FIG. 7.30 Gallbladder adenocarcinomas contain angulated glands lined by cells with neutral mucin and enlarged hyperchromatic nuclei.

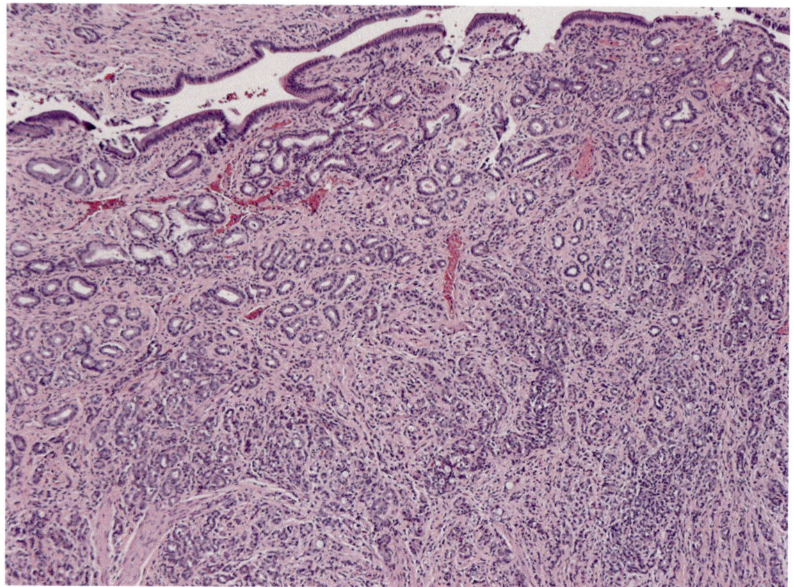

FIG. 7.31 Invasive adenocarcinoma fills the gallbladder mucosa. The surrounding stroma is inflamed, but not desmoplastic.

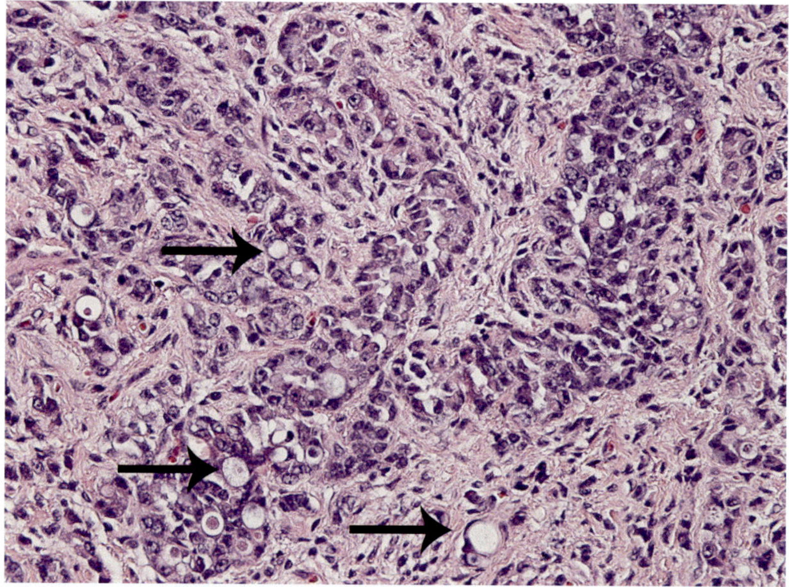

FIG. 7.32 Invasive adenocarcinoma in the gallbladder mucosa consists of inter-anastomosing glands with considerable cytologic atypia. Some mucin vacuoles are evident (*arrows*).

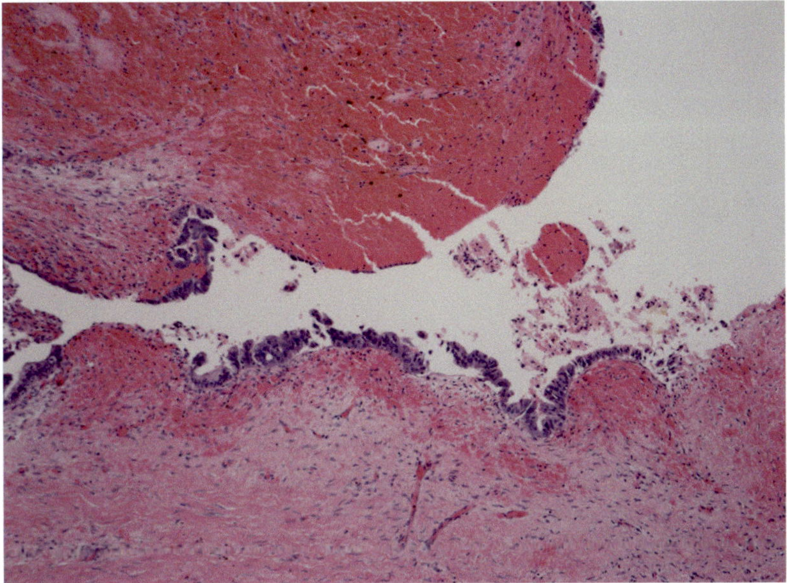

FIG. 7.33 The cystic duct margin is partially denuded in this resection specimen. However, the residual epithelium is atypical at low magnification.

sampling of the liver, omentum, or peritoneum for metastatic disease. Pathologic evaluation of the cystic duct margin may be problematic because invasive adenocarcinomas of the gallbladder colonize the cystic duct epithelium or are associated with dysplasia in the cystic duct (Figs. 7.33–7.36). Cancers may also spread in the cystic duct wall and show a predilection for perineural invasion. Frozen section analysis of the hepatic bed margin is generally straightforward since most gallbladder cancers are overtly malignant (Figs. 7.37 and 7.38). However, well-differentiated adenocarcinomas that involve the hepatic bed simulate aberrant ducts of Luschka. Distinguishing features of carcinoma include the haphazard arrangement of variably sized glands and their presence in all layers of the gallbladder wall, rather than linear proliferations of small ductules limited to adventitial or subserosal tissue (Figs. 7.39 and 7.40). Metastatic adenocarcinoma in the liver, omentum, or peritoneum is grossly similar to metastatic carcinoma from other sites. It produces one, or more firm white nodules comprised of infiltrating glands enmeshed in abundant collagenous stroma (Fig. 7.41).

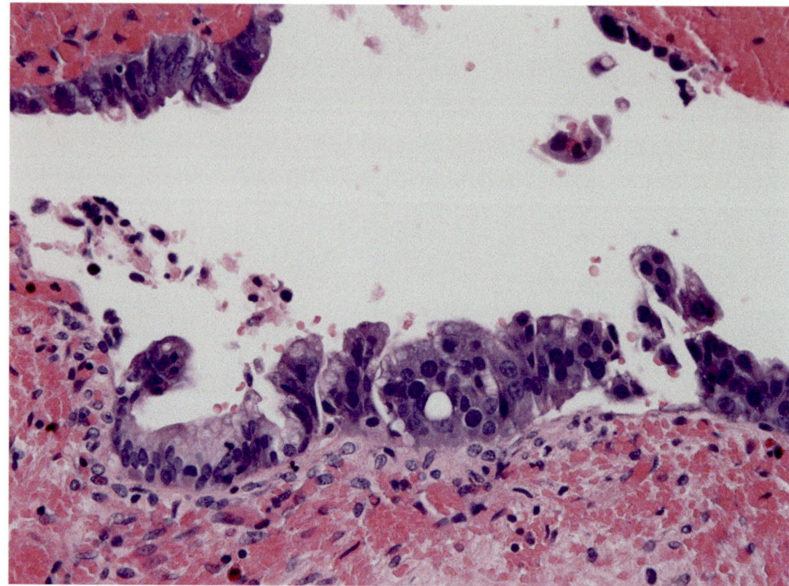

FIG. 7.34 Neoplastic epithelial cells are present at the cystic duct margin. This finding may represent epithelial dysplasia or colonization of the mucosa by the adjacent cancer (same case as Fig. 7.33).

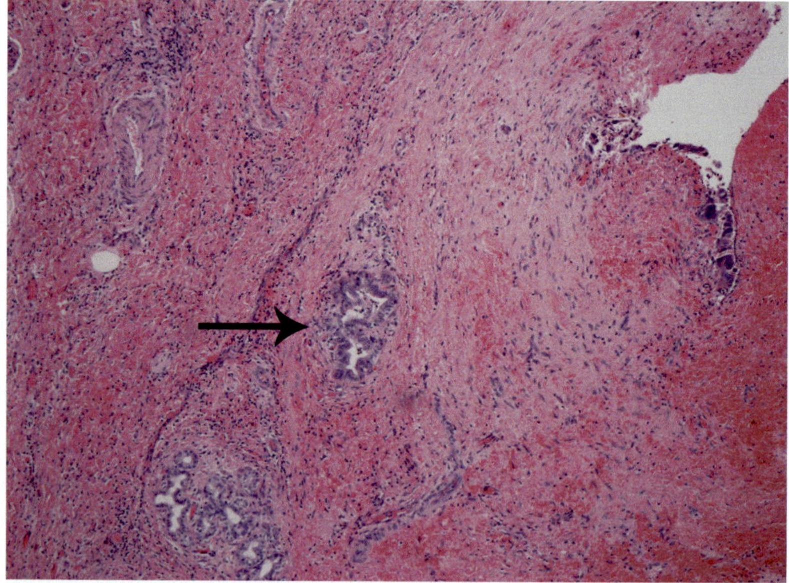

FIG. 7.35 A frozen section of the cystic duct from a patient with gallbladder adenocarcinoma shows aggregates of neoplastic glands in the wall (*arrow*).

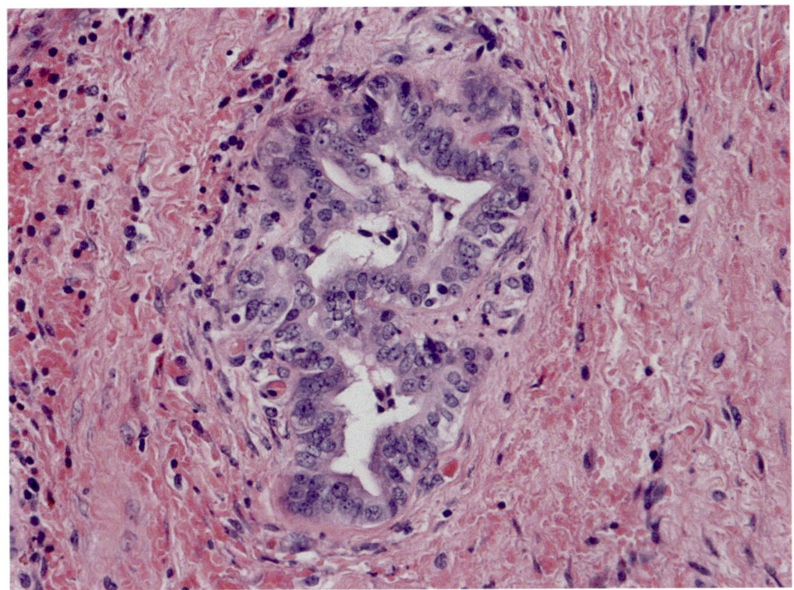

FIG. 7.36 Clusters of neoplastic glands are present in the wall of the cystic duct (same case as Fig. 7.35).

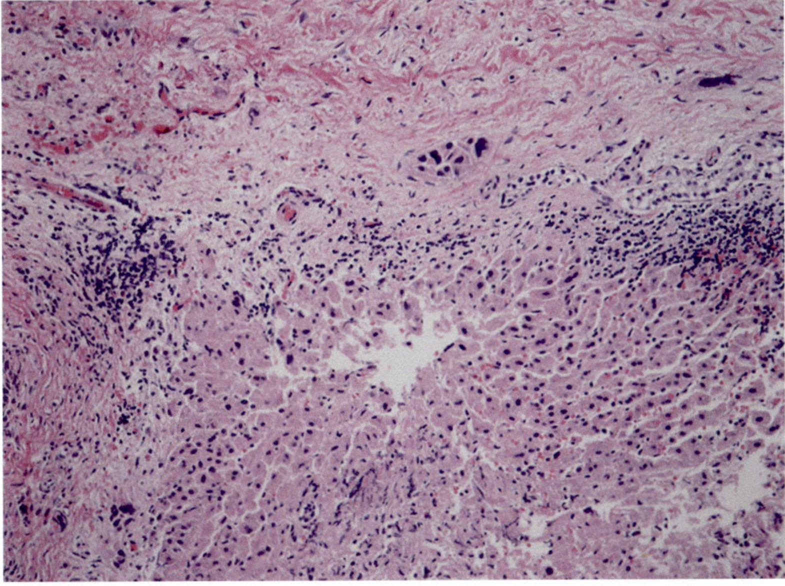

FIG. 7.37 Invasive adenocarcinoma in the hepatic bed contains irregularly shaped glands arranged in a haphazard fashion.

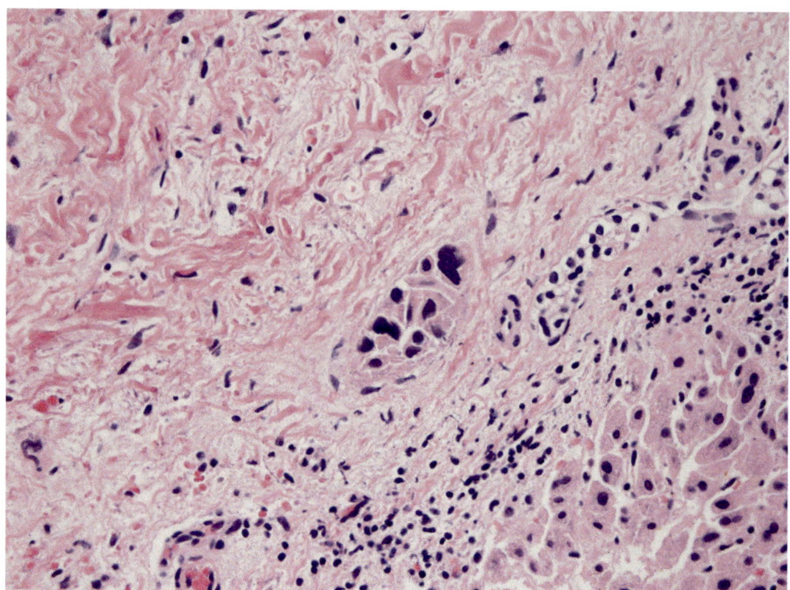

Fig. 7.38 The invasive glands contain overtly malignant cells with enlarged hyerpchromatic nuclei (same case as Fig. 7.37).

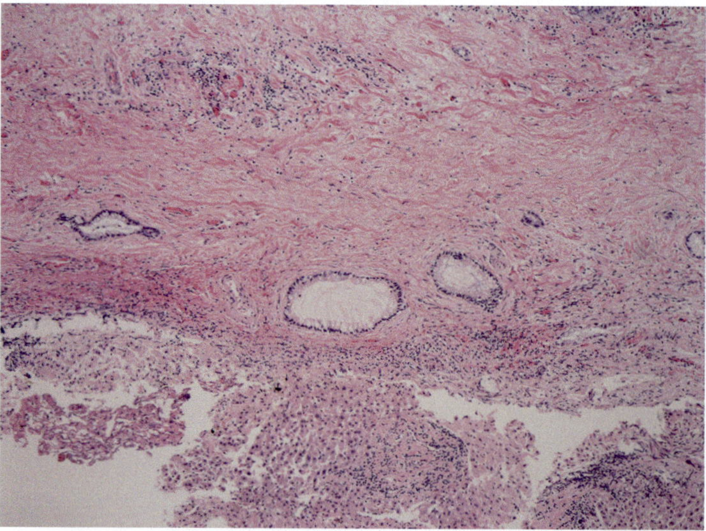

Fig. 7.39 Well-differentiated adenocarcinoma involving the hepatic bed consists of irregularly infiltrating glands of variable size. The surrounding stroma is desmoplastic.

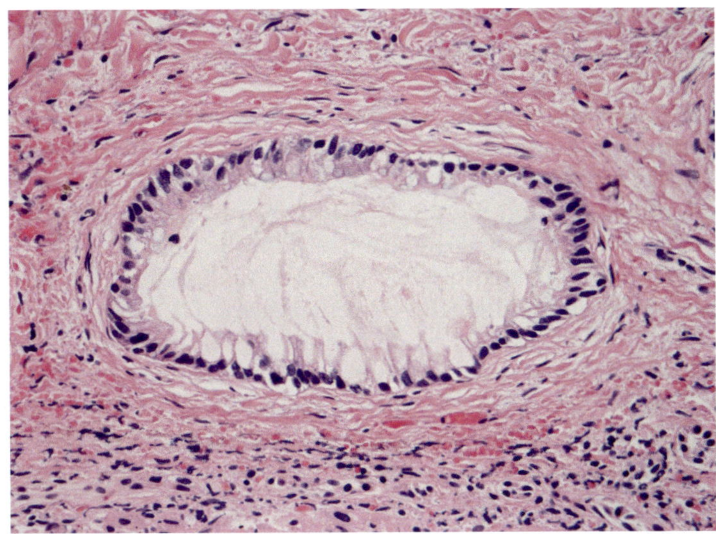

FIG. 7.40 The malignant glands of a gallbladder adenocarcinoma contain enlarged, hyperchromatic nuclei. Although the cells maintain their polarity, they show a greater degree of cytologic atypia than aberrant ducts (of Luschka). These features, in combination with cystic dilatation of glands and desmoplasia, are suggestive of malignancy (same case as Fig. 7.39).

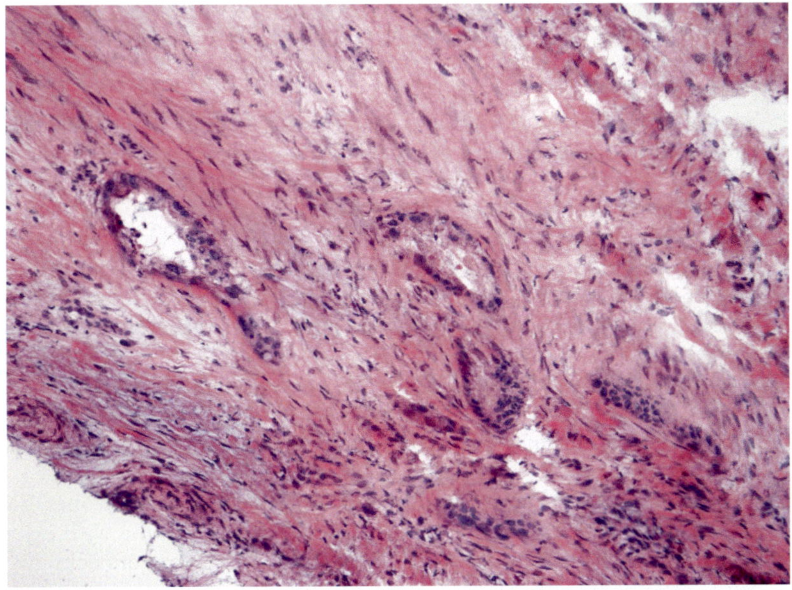

FIG. 7.41 Metastatic gallbladder adenocarcinoma in the peritoneal cavity produces multiple firm tan-white nodules comprised of infiltrating glands embedded in densely collagenous, or desmoplastic, stroma.

MESENCHYMAL TUMORS

Primary mesenchymal tumors of the gallbladder and biliary tract are uncommon, but benign and malignant tumors that show smooth muscle, adipose, vascular, and peripheral nerve sheath differentiation have been reported, as well as CD117-positive gastrointestinal stromal tumors [27]. Granular cell tumor is the most common benign mesenchymal tumor of the gallbladder. It is composed of cells with abundant eosinophilic, granular cytoplasm and small, uniform nuclei [28]. Primary malignant mesenchymal tumors of the gallbladder are extremely rare. Of these, embryonal rhabdomyosarcomas are probably the most frequent sarcomas and usually occur in young children under the age of 5 years [29]. These tumors are polypoid with a cambium layer of condensed sarcoma cells underlying benign epithelium. Frozen section analysis does not usually play an important role in the intraoperative evaluation of these tumors.

References

1. Weiland ST, Mahvi DM, Heisey DM, Chicks DS, Rikkers LF. Should suspected early gallbladder cancer be treated laparoscopically? J Gastrointest Surg. 2002;49(5):56–7.
2. Kwon AH, Imamura A, Kitade H, Kamiyama Y. Unsuspected gallbladder cancer diagnosed during or after laparoscopic cholecystectomy. J Surg Oncol. 2008;97(3):241–5.
3. Sun CD, Zhang BY, Wu LQ, Lee WJ. Laparoscopic cholecystectomy for treatment of unexpected early-stage gallbladder cancer. J Surg Oncol. 2005;91(4):253–7.
4. Sandri L, Colecchia A, Larocca A, et al. Gallbladder cholesterol polyps and cholesterolosis. Minerva Gastroenterol Dietol. 2003;49(3): 217–24.
5. Maeyama R, Yamaguchi K, Noshiro H, Takashima M, Chijiiwa K, Tanaka M. A large inflammatory polyp of the gallbladder masquerading as gallbladder carcinoma. J Gastroenterol. 1998;33(5):770–4.
6. Van Patten K, Jain D. Benign tumors and tumor-like lesions of the gallbladder and extrahepatic biliary tract. Diagn Histopathol. 2010; 16(8):371–9.
7. Spinelli A, Schumacher G, Pascher A, et al. Extended surgical resection for xanthogranulomatous cholecystitis mimicking advanced gallbladder carcinoma: a case report and review of literature. World J Gastroenterol. 2006;12(14):2293–6.
8. Pinocy J, Lange A, Konig C, Kaiserling E, Becker HD, Krober SM. Xanthogranulomatous cholecystitis resembling carcinoma with extensive tumorous infiltration of the liver and colon. Langenbecks Arch Surg. 2003;388(1):48–51.
9. Henderson JT, Yantiss RK. Non-neoplastic diseases of the gallbladder. Diagn Histopathol. 2010;16(8):350–9.

10. Albores-Saavedra J, Galliani C, Chable-Montero F, Batich K, Henson DE. Mucin-containing Rokitansky-Aschoff sinuses with extracelllar mucin deposits simulating mucinous carcinoma of the gallbladder. Am J Surg Pathol. 2009;33(11):1633–8.

11. Albores-Saavedra J, Keenportz B, Bejarano PA, Alexander AA, Henson DE. Adenomyomatous hyperplasia of the gallbladder with perineural invasion: revisited. Am J Surg Pathol. 2007;31(10):1598–604.

12. Adsay NV, Klimstra DS. Benign and malignant tumors of the gallbladder and extrahepatic biliary tree. In: Odze RD, Goldblum JR, editors. Surgical pathology of the GI tract, liver, biliary tract, and pancreas. Philadelphia: Saunders Elsevier; 2009. p. 845–75.

13. Albores-Saavedra J, Adsay NV, Crawford JM, et al. Tumours of the gallbladder and extrahepatic biliary tree. In: Bosman FT, Carneiro F, Hruban RH, Theise ND, editors. WHO classification of tumours of the digestive system. 4th ed. Lyon: IARC Press; 2010. p. 263–76.

14. Mastoraki A, Papanikolaou IS, Konstandidadou I, Sakorafas G, Safioleas M. Facing the challenge of treating gallbladder carcinoma review of the literature. Hepatogastroenterology. 2010;57(98):215–9.

15. Towfigh S, McFadden DW, Cortina G, et al. Porcelain gallbladder is not associated with gallbladder carcinoma. Am Surg. 2001;67(1):7–10.

16. Walsh N, Qizilbash A, Banerjee R, Waugh GA. Biliary neoplasia in Gardner's syndrome. Arch Pathol Lab Med. 1987;111(1):76–7.

17. Mekeel KL, Hemming AW. Surgical managment of gallbladder carcinoma: a review. J Gastrointest Surg. 2007;11(9):1188–93.

18. Reid KM, Ramos-De la Medina A, Donohue JH. Diagnosis and surgical management of gallbladder cancer: a review. J Gastrointest Surg. 2007;11(5):671–81.

19. Eguchi H, Ishikawa O, Ohigashi H, et al. Surgical significance of superficial cancer spread in early gallbladder cancer. Jpn J Clin Oncol. 2005;35(3):134–8.

20. Shirai Y, Wakai T, Hatakeyama K. Radical lymph node dissection for gallbladder cancer: indications and limitations. Surg Oncol Clin N Am. 2007;16(1):221–32.

21. Yamaguchi K, Chijiiwa K, Saiki S, Shimizu S, Tsuneyoshi M, Tanaka M. Reliability of frozen section diagnosis of gallbladder tumor for detecting carcinoma and depth of invasion. J Surg Oncol. 1997;65:132–6.

22. Lai CH, Lau WY. Aggressive surgical resection for carcinoma of gallbladder. ANZ J Surg. 2005;75(6):441–4.

23. De Aretxabala X, Roa I, Hepp J, et al. Early gallbladder cancer: is further treatment necessary? J Surg Oncol. 2009;100(7):589–93.

24. Steinert R, Nestler G, Sagynaliev E, Muller J, Lippert H, Reymond MA. Laparoscopic cholecytectomy and gallbladder cancer. J Surg Oncol. 2006;93(8):682–9.

25. Yildirim E, Celen O, Gulben K, Berberoglu U. The surgical management of incidental gallbladder carcinoma. Eur J Surg Oncol. 2005;31(1):45–52.

26. Pilgrim C, Usatoff V, Evans PM. A review of surgical strategies for the management of gallbladder carcinoma based on T stage and growth type of the tumour. Eur J Surg Oncol. 2009;35(9):903–7.

27. Peerlinck ID, Irvin TT, Sarsfield PT, Harington JM. GIST (gastro-intestinal stromal tumour) of the gallbladder: a case report. Acta Chir Belg. 2004;104(1):107–9.
28. Murakata LA, Ishak KG. Expression of inhibin-alpha by granular cell tumors of the gallbladder and extrahepatic bile ducts. Am J Surg Pathol. 2001;25(9):1200–3.
29. Al-Daraji WI, Makhlouf HR, Miettinen M, et al. Primary gallbladder sarcoma: a clinicopathologic study of 15 cases, heterogeneous sarcoma with poor outcome, except pediatric botryoid rhabdomyosarcoma. Am J Surg Pathol. 2009;33(6):826–34.

Index

R.K. Yantiss (ed.), *Frozen Section Library: Liver, Extrahepatic Biliary Tree
and Gallbladder*, Frozen Section Library, DOI 10.1007/978-1-4614-0043-1,
© Springer Science+Business Media, LLC 2011

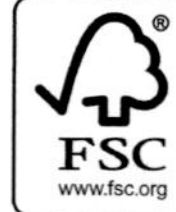

MIX
Papier aus verantwortungsvollen Quellen
Paper from responsible sources
FSC® C105338

If you have any concerns about our products,
you can contact us on
ProductSafety@springernature.com

In case Publisher is established outside the EU,
the EU authorized representative is:
Springer Nature Customer Service Center GmbH
Europaplatz 3, 69115 Heidelberg, Germany

Printed by Libri Plureos GmbH
in Hamburg, Germany